HEAL

YOURSELF!

Discover quantum healing energy, attract
miracles and good luck in 3 easy steps

Dr. Alexander Khomoutov, Ph.D.

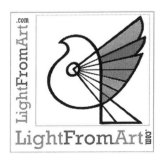

LightFromArt.com

Dr. Alexander Khomoutov, Ph.D.

ISBN: 1979904782

ISBN-13: 978-1979904780

We are in an auspicious time on the planet. It is a time where the essential nature of human consciousness is evolving in profound ways. We are entering into a new reality – one that includes an awareness of our personal spiritual power, and the energetic nature of life. With this change – many people are learning to work with their energy fields to promote healing and wellbeing in unconventional ways. In this book Alexander takes you on a journey, a personal one, where he shares with you what he learned – in his own experience of healing.

In these pages, Alexander shares with you how he discovered not only his "spiritual DNA" but also the power to heal through conscious communication with it! Using kinesiology and other healing practices – he was able to talk to his body and his DNA – and learn innately what was helpful to support him in healing. Although it may sound too mystical to be true – this can be done – and Alexander is one of the pioneers who is using this information in a powerful way for healing and transformation.

Let Alexander's experience inspire you! Every human being has this power - and so do You! The time is now upon us to learn to use it! Enjoy this story of love and healing. May it open a window that allows you to expand what you think is possible – when you dare to dream!

Dr. John G. Ryan, MD
Specialist Medical Doctor, consciousness and energy based healer, University Professor, Author of The Missing Pill, and Harp of the One Heart – Poetic words of Ascension.

Dr. Alexander Khomoutov, Ph.D.

One of the things I liked about Dr. Khomoutov's book is that he describes in detail, exactly the steps he takes to effect healing change. If he is talking about foods or herbs he used, he tells exactly what he used, how it was prepared, and when and under what circumstances he used it. This is his own personal story of how he healed himself, and as such, he chronicles how he progressed over a period of time, often like daily log entries, so that the reader can do something similar if he/she chooses. He also shares some of the methods his wife, Elena, uses, and what has worked for her.

He is very forthright and clear about all the methods he uses, where he learned about the methods, and including some special "tweaks" he has used to enhance what works for him but always being careful to say what might or might not work in your own case. He leaves it up to you to pick the methods that might work best for you, based on the choices and options he puts forth.

I also liked his reference to his budgie, Gosha, whom he describes as "our family angel," and the message Gosha brought to Alexander and Elena. Having had beloved pet birds myself, I could very much relate to the love they felt for Gosha and how deeply Gosha's sudden passing must have affected them and how important and urgent Gosha's message became.

The methods and practices Alexander speaks of in this book may take time to implement. Isn't loving ourselves first and caring about ourselves more the main message that Gosha's passing was meant to convey worth our time, if it can bring us amazing healing, good luck, love and unlock the miraculous power within us to live a healthy, happy and joyful life? The miracle of working with Spiritual DNA, the higher power within you, can have profound effects even with other problems, like (in Elena's case) ants in the garden, or many different aspects of your life.

This is a truly spiritually-infused writing, and I am sure the teachings and methods of healing the author puts forth in this book can be of great insight and benefit to anyone who is open enough to put them into practice.

Dr. Marcy Rae Lifavi, D.C., C.Ht.
Doctor of Chiropractic, Certified Hypnotherapist,
Artist and Author of Eletunji, The Shiny Elephant:
A Fable: Spiritual And Psychological Journey Creates Choice for A Nurturing Voice.

In this book the author shares his personal struggle to heal his own body from unexplained pain.
On his journey he learns a number of techniques that enable him to connect with his Spiritual DNA guidance.

"How to Heal Yourself" will give the readers tremendous insights into how our subconscious mind can be a guiding force leading us down the path of making good positive decisions about our health, happiness, and wellbeing.

Dr. Alexander Khomoutov, Ph.D.

Dianne Nassr, L.C. M.S.W.
An energy healer and contributing author of the
book A Juicy, Joyful Life: Inspiration from Women
Who Have Found the Sweetness in Every Day.

Dedication

This book is dedicated to my wife Elena and angel Gosha. They inspired me to write this book.

The book is dedicated to all of you who are open to discovering the power within yourselves to live a happy, joyful and healthy life ever after...

Dr. Alexander Khomoutov, Ph.D.

Table of Contents

Get Alexander Khomoutov's 7 gifts FOR FREE

Alexander creates his art, photographs and books with the intention of bringing you healing energy and good luck.

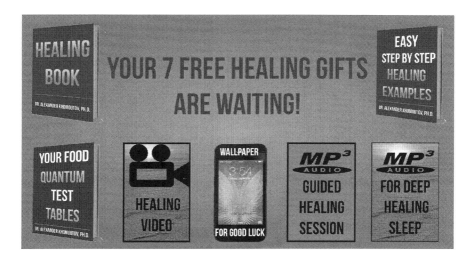

Get Alexander's 7 healing gifts:
- Healing book
- Easy step by step healing examples
- Your food quantum test tables
- Good luck energy wallpaper for your iPhone / Android devices
- Healing video
- 2 healing audio files

All free when you join his Reader's Group.

Find details at the end of this book.

Acknowledgments

Thank you to my wife Elena. She inspired me to write this book and she was the first reader, who gave me so many suggestions.

I'm so thankful to my parents, who gave me the freedom to do what I love. They always trusted that I would use this freedom in a very positive and loving way. Very special thanks to my mother who showed me how to use the greatest power within. In 1960s and-70s she was already successfully using applied kinesiology – using a pendulum —to determine blood pressure and other things.

I'm very grateful to Lee Carroll and Kryon. Their teachings about the Innate inspired me. They gave me a magic key to unlock the sacred door to my healing and joy.

I'd like to express my very special thanks to Dr. John G. Ryan MD whose book "The Missing Pill" gave me deeper understanding of Spiritual/Quantum DNA.

I'm so grateful to Dianne Nassr. Dianne taught me how to use Sway test when I was hosting "Healing with Lightworkers" telesummit. This is the main method I use now. She also gave me numerous suggestions to improve the book.

I'm so thankful to Janet Hofstetter for a great copy editing.

I'm very grateful to you my dear Spiritual/Quantum DNA for healing, love, joy and happiness. You were so patient to wait so long before I connected to you for the first time ☺.

I'm sending to all of you my Love, Light and Hugs.

Alexander Khomoutov

Disclaimer

The author of this book does not dispense medical advice or prescribe the use of any technique as a form of diagnosis or treatment for physical, emotional or medical problems without advice of a physician, either directly or indirectly. The intent of the author is only to offer information of a general nature to help you in your quest for emotional and spiritual well-being.

Please also be informed that any artworks, images, information from this book, etc. are not intended to diagnose, treat, cure or prevent any condition, including: physical, financial or any other problems. The information received through any of these means should not in any way be used as a substitute for advice from a Medical Advisor or other licensed Professionals.

In the event you use any of the information in this book for yourself, the author and the publisher assume no responsibility for your actions.

Introduction

Do you want to discover how to heal yourself? You're in the right place, because these easy effective 3 steps take only few minutes to learn now and can be used instantly!

Did you have any pain? I had a big moving pain in my chest almost every night for 8 months. It was so strong that I couldn't sleep. I was getting weaker and weaker every day and felt that I was going to die. As you read this book, I'll talk about the sudden death of an angel in our family — our budgie, Gosha — and how that became the turning point in my life and showed me the way to heal myself.

Finally, after 8 months of struggles, I found a very easy solution that worked miraculously for me. And I am sharing my discoveries with you in this book.

It's not just a book, it is positive energy tool to help you. A good luck energy deeply embedded in every page of the book.

Thank you to everyone who gave me great feedback on my first edition of How to Heal Yourself. I've used that feedback to make many improvements and additions, including:

- A new Questions and Answers chapter
- An example of how to use the tables in the Appendix to find the foods that will heal you and the ones you should avoid. I also revised the tables.
- New methods of communicating with your Quantum DNA:
  - pendulum method
  - L-shaped indicators method
- An image for the shifting energy ball method.

The book was written with intention of helping you attract good luck energy to support your healing. Just by reading this book you are already in the good luck quantum field, if you open your heart for it. The choice is always yours.

Your first step is to read this book in its entirety. Please don't just skim through it. I don't want you to miss a single word, because it has healing energy...

1. How it started

Early in 2014, my wife and I were preparing for a 3-week trip to Europe. I was so nervous and busy that I didn't pay attention to the chest pain that I was experiencing at night. I just tried to sleep with it. But just ignoring it didn't help at all. The pain became stronger and stronger. It was a very unusual, moving pain. One day it could be in one place, and the next day in another. Sometimes it moved around my chest and then it might move to my belly. By June, I couldn't sleep at all when I felt it. When I felt the pain in the middle of the night, I reached for a drink of some healing herbal tea with honey and tried to do some work on the computer until the pain stopped. Sometimes it was more than 2 hours before I could fall asleep again. But I kept up my busy schedule. I thought that a 3 km run in the morning, some healing herbal tea and good healthy food would be enough to remedy the pains I was experiencing. But those things didn't work.

I was regularly sending Good Luck energy, Love and healing hugs to my Facebook community, but I didn't take time to heal myself.

Suddenly, our family's angel, a budgie named Gosha, developed a problem with his eye. He couldn't even open it. I sent him a healing energy and asked my Facebook friends to help him. Many of them sent prayers and healing energy to him, and Gosha's eye healed quite quickly.

But I didn't ask my Facebook friends to help me. And I didn't take the time to heal myself either.

Gosha's eye was healed, but my pains became stronger and stronger. I slept less and less at night, and I became weaker and weaker.

July arrived. Time for our trip to Europe. I experienced pain during the sleepless night before we left for our trip and the next day while doing some final preparations. It continued on the long, sleepless flight to Europe and was still with me throughout that very busy first day.

I went more than 48 hours without sleep. It was a very tough time. The next 3 weeks were exciting, full of interesting events and meetings, but still I was not getting enough sleep. The pains moving in my body woke me up in the night again and again.

Every week I was sending LIGHT & Love and healing energy and Good Luck to thousands of my Facebook friends, but I didn't take time to send Love to myself.

I did not have my usual energy, and this had a detrimental effect on our art sales. That made me anxious and fearful, which made my condition even worse. After 3 weeks of vacation, I returned home exhausted, and my pains became even stronger.

2. First attempts to heal myself

When I came back from the trip my health was very poor. My night pain had become chronic and I was 6 kg below my normal weight. I realized I needed to spend time looking after myself. I started a new routine of positive affirmations, exercise, and healthy eating.

I would repeat these positive affirmations out aloud first thing in the morning:

I'm safe

I'm happy

I'm healthy

I'm at ease

And so it is.

I started a routine of running two to three kilometers before breakfast every morning.

I made a special herbal tea with mint, chamomile, Saint-John's-wort, valerian root, ground fennel seeds, Echinacea and honey. I drank some whenever I had some pain and about 1.5 liters during the day between meals. I made sure I ate only healthy foods.

I also started to use a special device that I built myself for energy balancing. It sends electric pulses to acupuncture points.

These healing steps had helped me in the past. But this time, after a week, there was no improvement.

I was scared. I called my family doctor. The secretary asked me about my symptoms and set up an appointment. The next day I got a phone call from the doctor's office recommending that I go directly to the hospital.

I didn't want to go there. I remembered how I had spent a half a day at the hospital waiting in line with bleeding wounds after a bicycle accident. I decided, instead, to seek the help of a professional energy healer.

3. Help from an energy healer

In the middle of August, I decided to find a good energy healer. I love the wonderful book, "Energy Medicine", by Donna Eden [1]. I decided to find a local practitioner who uses Donna's energy healing techniques. On the Internet I found a local practitioner. She had learned from Donna, and was certified by her to perform energy healing. A few days later I had a very helpful 90-minute energy session that helped me a lot. After that session, I had a good night's sleep for the first time in months. I was so happy. But this success was temporary. In a few weeks, the pains came back.

I understood that only by using my inner power could I cure myself. And I have to cure the root of the problem so it won't come back.

4. Experimentation with different healing approaches

From September 2014 to February 2015 I tried many things to heal myself. Sometimes things went well for few days, even a week, but then the night pains would return. Until I found a miraculous cure. Keep reading. You'll find out soon.

4.1 Innate, Quantum DNA method

Usually scientists talk about DNA from a biochemical point of view without considering the biophysical characteristics. According to esoteric teachings, DNA has also vibrational, quantum nature. Some people call it Quantum DNA, Spiritual DNA, Soul DNA or Innate. Find more about Spiritual DNA at Dr. John Ryan's book "The Missing Pill" [6].

From Lee Carol's channelings of Kryon [2, 3] I found that we can reprogram our DNA for a long, healthy life by communicating with the Quantum DNA.

So I meditated, connected to my Quantum DNA and

asked to reprogram it to be healthy and balanced to provide a long life with active evolution. In spite of this, the pain came back on some nights. Maybe I wasn't connected properly, when I was doing the reprogramming? I thought. Later in the book you will find out how to check the connection with your Quantum DNA.

On the 7th of January 2015 I realized that it could be something I had inherited from my father who had similar problems. So I meditated, connected to Quantum DNA and asked to reprogram my DNA to make me free from inherited problems.

On the 9th of January during my 5 km run, I caught myself thinking about the past and the future but not enjoying the beautiful sunny day right here in the present moment.

I switched my awareness. I felt the fresh air energizing me. I felt joy. Joy shone from inside and out of me, and when I returned I was in the NOW. I got an internal strong message that I didn't need to go anywhere to be joyful. My joy is always inside me and ready to come out, just waiting to be invited to my NOW.

On 11th of January I had the following conversation with my Quantum DNA. I know that it's hard to believe, but try to be open. I used an applied kinesiology method to communicate to my Quantum DNA. Read on to find out how.

4.2 Applied Kinesiology (AK) or muscle testing techniques

George J. Goodheart, a chiropractor, pioneered an applied kinesiology technique in 1964 and began teaching it to other chiropractors [4]. While this practice is primarily used by chiropractors, it is also used by other practitioners now, for example in treating allergies [5]. People are sometimes skeptical about whether it will work until they've tried it themselves and see the results. Applied kinesiology, sometimes called a muscle testing technique, is a way to get information from the subconscious.

There are several techniques available. Some methods that you can use to test yourself include:

- Hole-In-One Method
- Linked Rings Method
- Shifting Energy Ball Method
- Dowsing Method using L-shaped rods
- Pendulum method
- Sway Test

I tried several of these methods over a period of 6 months to find one with most consistent results. I found one method that works very well for me – the sway test. I learned it from Dianne Nassr when I was hosting the "Healing with Lightworkers" telesummit [11]. The telesummit was packed with amazing healing information, but this method changed my life. Since that time, I have used mostly this method because I find it gives me the most reliable results. I will show you how to use sway test and other methods. Read on to find out how.

4.3 Using the sway test

The sway test is one of the best and simplest methods to get answers from your subconscious mind, Spiritual DNA and Higher Self. It doesn't require the assistance of anyone else. You must be standing to use it (see fig.1), and it takes a bit more time than the other self-testing methods.

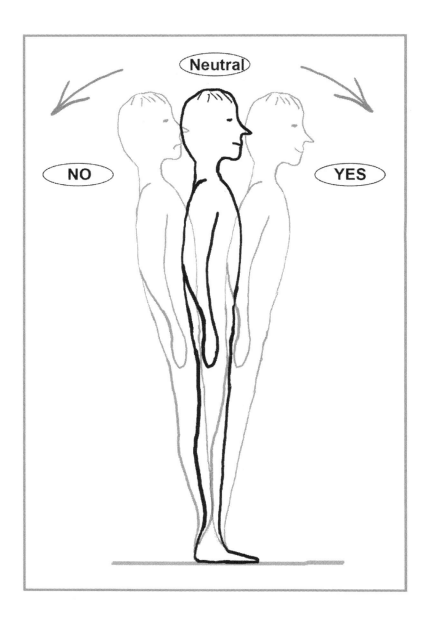

Fig. 1. Sway test.

Preparation

Use the following steps to prepare for the sway test:

1. Go to a quiet room free of distractions like music or television. For me, it works the best when I'm alone in the room, but you could do it with somebody else who is willing to do it with you.

2. Stand still, with your feet shoulder width apart for a good balance and your hands at your sides.

   Some descriptions of this method recommend that you face north, but in my experience I find that it works equally well facing in any direction.

3. Let go of all worries and relax your body. If you are comfortable doing so, close your eyes. If you find it difficult to balance with your eyes closed, doing it with open eyes is OK too.

4. Imagine that golden white light beam connects 3 points in your body: the heart, the heart chakra, and the crown chakra. See fig.2.

   This is my own addition to the standard method. If you are just starting to practice the sway method, you could skip this point, but I find that if I do it, I have more consistent results.

5. Use a hand finger gesture while imagining the beam of light (step 4). (This is another one of my additions to the standard method, and it is optional.) Slowly bunch your fingertips together, with tips touching and pointing upward. See fig.4. You could do it with your left or right hand or with both hands at the same time. I prefer to do this with both hands at the same time.

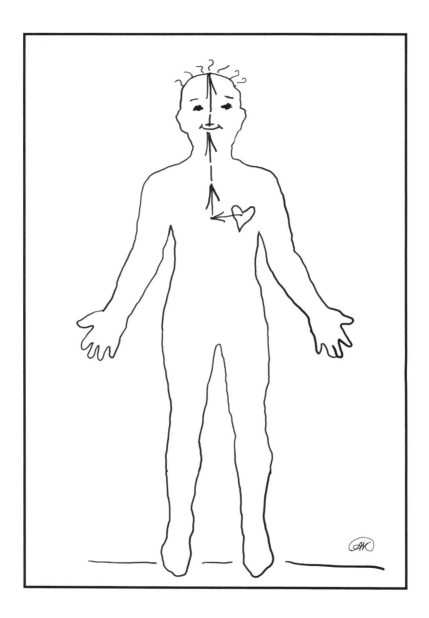

Fig.2. I imagine a golden white light beam connects 3 points: my heart, the heart chakra, and the crown chakra.

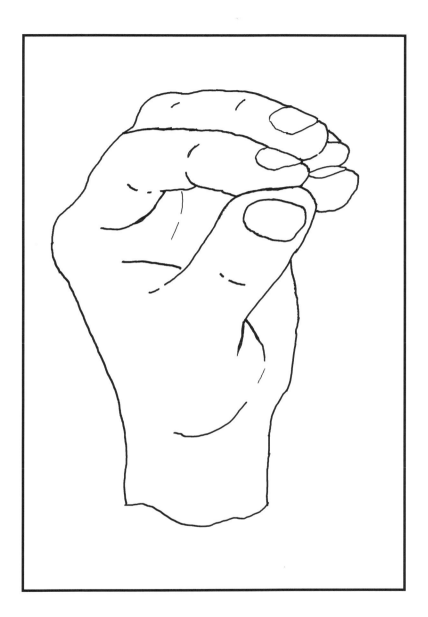

Fig.3. Gesture of balance.

For me, this hand gesture symbolizes connection with Quantum DNA and balance. I found that with practice I can do just this gesture to establish a connection with my Quantum DNA almost instantly. If you are just starting to practice the sway method, you could skip it.

Alternatively, you could use another gesture or mudra, for example, the Gyan Mudra, known as the mudra of knowledge. See fig.4. Touch the tip of the thumb to the tip of the index finger, with the other three fingers stretched out. This mudra increases memory power and sharpens the brain. It also enhances concentration and prevents insomnia. Some people also use it as OK gesture. Notice that your body continually shifts its position very slightly in different directions as your muscles work to keep your balance. The movements are subtle, barely noticeable, because they aren't under your conscious control.

Perform the sway test

Perform the sway test using these steps:

1. Make a conscious attempt to communicate with your Quantum DNA. Say aloud, "I'm connected to my Quantum DNA."

2. To test that you have a connection, state aloud something that you know that is 100% true, for example, "My name is <your name>". In my case, I say "My name is Alexander".

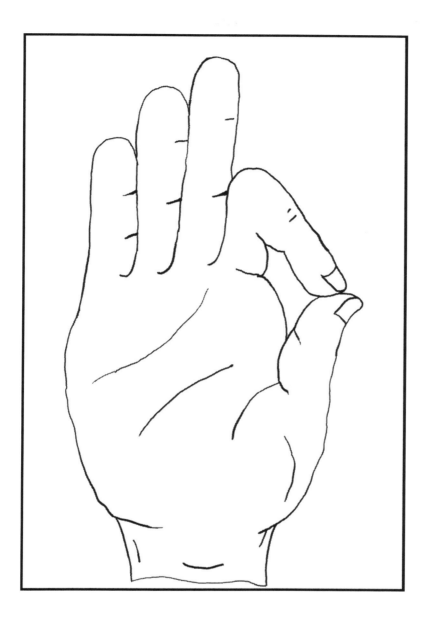

Fig.4. Gyan Mudra – mudra of knowledge.

You are giving your subconscious mind, Quantum DNA a chance to speak to you in this way. Your subconscious mind, Quantum DNA knows what is true. When you make a true statement, your body leans forward, because your body is drawn towards positivity and truth. Your body should begin to lean noticeably forward, usually within a few seconds. It means YES.

3. Continue testing the connection with your Quantum DNA. Make an untrue statement, for an example "my name is <somebody's name>". In my case I say "My name is Elena". As long as you choose a name that isn't yours, your subconscious mind will know that this statement is untrue. Your body will lean backwards within a few seconds. It means NO.

4. Say "Neutral" to have your body come back to the neutral position. I do this between any questions. This is my own addition to the standard method. I find that it makes results more reliable.

5. Repeat the true or false tests described in the previous steps several times in random order to make sure that you are getting reliable results before asking the main question for which you seek an answer.

6. State "I'm connected to my Quantum DNA". Your body should begin to lean noticeably forward, usually within a few seconds. It means that you are ready to communicate with your Quantum DNA.

7. Now you are ready to ask your main question. Ask your question in a way that can be answered with just "Yes" or "No." Then if your body leans forward the answer is "Yes," but if it leans backwards then the answer is "No."

Some tips for getting more reliable responses:

- Allow your body to sway on its own. Don't force it. Be patient! Practice every day with questions to which you know the answers already. When you'll have reliable answers then you are ready to ask some other questions. Your body's response time will shorten significantly after you practice every day for several weeks.

- When you ask questions, keep your mind clear of other thoughts. Stay focused on the question you are asking. If your thoughts are wandering, it will be difficult for your subconscious mind, your Spiritual DNA, to determine exactly what you are really asking. What if, for example, after your question you immediately begin thinking about the argument you had with somebody today? You'll probably sway backwards because the memory of that event is negative, and your body will naturally want to move away from it.

- If you are planning to ask many questions or your testing is taking more time than usual, it's a good idea to recheck your baseline periodically. Use a question for which you know the correct answer, for example your name and somebody else's name. If you get the right response, then continue your session.

- Allow love to fill your heart. Do not think about yourself negatively.

- Prepare your questions carefully. The wording of the question has to be exact. Ensure they questions can be answered with "Yes" or "No".

- Be sure that you are hydrated! Drinking a glass of

water 15-20 minutes before the session will be very useful.

Do you want to try this method? I will give you an example how I do it and then you will try it on your own.

I initiate connection as described above in the chapter 1.4.3. I always test the connection first as the following:

> *Me: I'm connected to my Quantum DNA.*
> *Quantum DNA: Yes.*
> *Me: I'm Alexander.*
> *Quantum DNA: Yes.*
> *Me: Neutral.*
> *Me: I'm <somebody's name, for example Peter>.*
> *Quantum DNA: No.*

Sometimes I do this test several times to make sure that I'm really connected. I always test the connection before any communications, so I'll be skipping the description of the test for the rest of the book.

- I had the following conversation with my Quantum DNA.

> *Me: Dear Quantum DNA, is a mint tea good for me?*
> *Quantum DNA: Yes.*
> *Me: Thank you.*

Now try to use the above example.

See pros and cons of using the sway method below.

Pros:

- It's easy to learn.

- It can be used in public places without anybody noticing it.

Cons:

- You have to stand to use it.

- For some people it's not possible to use if they have body balancing issues or problems with their spine.

- It takes more time than most of the other methods.

If for any reason you can't use the sway method, try the other methods listed in section 4.2 and described in sections 4.4 through 4.6. Try them until you find the one that is most suitable and reliable for you.

4.4 Pendulum method

I was introduced to this method when I was 16 years old. My mother has shown me how she measures a blood pressure using the pendulum method. But this is also a good method to find artworks with positive energies as well.

When my mother showed me how to use it I was very impressed. She was using just 2 things: a small wooden metric ruler 200 mm (about 8 inches) long, and her wedding ring on a string used as a pendulum. See fig.5.C. That's it. She put the ruler on my left hand and moved the pendulum along the ruler slowly from 0 mm to 150 mm. The ring was very close to the ruler, but not touching it. The ring started swinging across the ruler. At first, it vibrated at about 65 mm and then she moved it further and the pendulum became quiet again. The ring started swinging side to side across the ruler again when it reached about 115 mm. She then moved the pendulum further and the pendulum became quiet again. So the blood pressure was about 115 systolic and 65 diastolic, read as "115 over 65".

These blood pressure numbers are for demonstration purposes only. I don't remember the exact numbers, because it was so long ago, but they were very similar. Later, when I finished my studies at the university and started to work, I bought a gift for my mother's birthday – a standard device to measure blood pressure. It was the same blood pressure cuff that the local doctors were using.

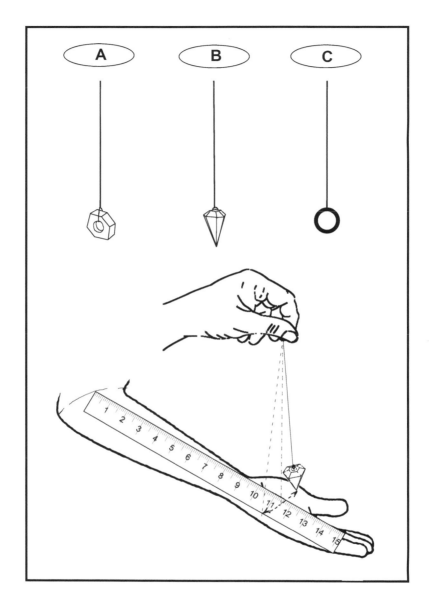

Fig.5. Pendulum method

We then ran a comparison test. Do you think that we acquired different results? Actually, the results were very close! From that point on, I have successfully used my mother's method for a long time and I haven't need to buy any devices for myself. Only recently, I bought one for my wife and ran a comparison test again. I have listed the results below.

Usually the pendulum consist of a crystal attached to a string. See fig.5.B. In this situation I made a pendulum using just a simple small metal nut and string. See fig.5.A. I measured my blood pressure using the pendulum and got 65 / 110. Then I used a special electronic device to measure it and got 67 / 100. I removed the device then put it on again and measured 65/100.

I repeated the test the following day.

Elena tried to measure her blood pressure this morning and got an error message. I recharged the batteries and tried to measure my blood pressure using the metal nut pendulum method again: 70/120 and with device: 70/100 and the second time the device readings were 69/100. Then I used the pendulum with a small crystal ball and got 70/105. It looks like the crystal ball pendulum worked better for me than the metal nut pendulum.

Personally, I prefer to use the electronic device. I've done this experiment just to test that this method works for me. I could use it to communicate with my Quantum DNA and get some other answers that are not related to my blood pressure. Ask your Quantum DNA to give you the "Yes" answer by swinging the pendulum back and forth, and the "No" answer when the pendulum is swinging from side to side. See fig.6.A and fig.6.B accordingly. Some people have better results for "YES" – the pendulum is swinging clockwise and then it will swing counterclockwise for "NO." So, choose whatever method works for you even if it is contrary to what I have described.

This method is very easy to use to find what artwork will bring positive energy. Continue reading to find examples of this technique.

Preparation

Use the following steps to prepare for the pendulum method:

1. Go to a quiet room free of distractions like music or television.

   For me, it works the best when I'm alone in the room, but you could do it with somebody else who is willing to do it with you.

2. Stand still, with your feet shoulder width apart for good balance and holding the pendulum in your one hand. See Fig.6. You could do it also when you are sitting.

3. Let go of all worries and relax your body.

4. Imagine that a golden-white light beam connects 3 points in your body: the heart, the heart chakra, and the crown chakra. See fig.2.

   This is my own addition to the standard method. If you are just starting to practice the pendulum method, you could skip this point, but I find that if I do it, I have more consistent results.

5. With the hand not holding the pendulum, make a hand finger gesture while imagining the beam of light (step 4). (This is another one of my additions to the standard method, and it is optional.) Slowly bunch your fingertips together, with tips touching and pointing upward. See fig.3.

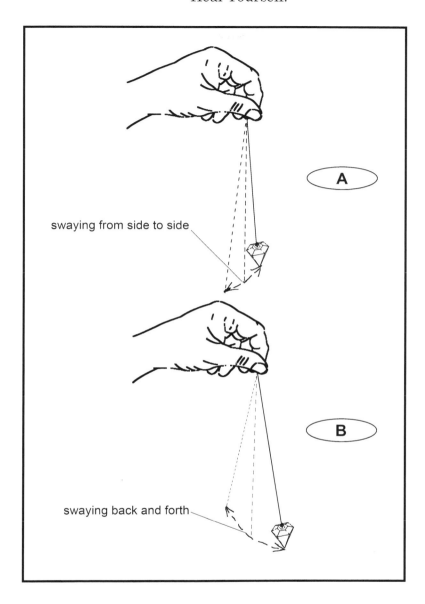

Fig.6. Pendulum method

Perform the pendulum method

Perform the pendulum method using these steps:

1. Make a conscious attempt to communicate with your Quantum DNA. Say aloud, "I'm connected to my Quantum DNA."

2. To test that you have a connection, state aloud something that you know that is 100% true, for example, "My name is <your name>". In my case, I say "My name is Alexander".

   You are giving your subconscious mind, your Quantum DNA, a chance to speak to you in this way. Your Quantum DNA knows what is true. When you make a true statement, your pendulum begins to swing back and forth noticeably, perpendicular to your body, usually within a few seconds. It means YES. See fig.6.

3. Continue testing the connection with your Quantum DNA. Make an untrue statement, for example "my name is <somebody's name>". In my case I say "My name is Elena". As long as you choose a name that isn't yours, your subconscious mind will know that this statement is untrue. Your pendulum will begin to swing side to side noticeably, parallel to your body, usually within a few seconds. It means NO. See fig.6.

4. Say "Neutral" to have your pendulum stop oscillating. Do this in between your questions. I find that it makes the results more reliable.

5. Repeat the true or false tests described in the previous steps several times in random order to make sure that you are getting reliable results before asking the main question for which you seek an answer.

6. State "I'm connected to my Quantum DNA".

Your pendulum begins to swing noticeably back and force, usually within a few seconds. It means that you are ready to communicate with your Quantum DNA.

7. Say "Neutral" to have your pendulum stop swinging.

8. Now you are ready to ask your main question. Ask your question in a way that can be answered with just "Yes" or "No." Then, if your pendulum begins to swing noticeably back and forth, the answer is "Yes," but if it swings from side to side then your answer is "No."

See pros and cons of using this method below.

Pros:

- It's easy to learn
- You may sit or stand to use it
- Fast results

Cons:

- Not easy to use in public places without drawing attention to yourself
- For some people, it's not possible to use if they have any problems with their hand.

If for any reason you can't use the pendulum method, try the other methods described in chapter 4. Try them until you find the one that is most suitable and reliable for you.

4.5 Dowsing method, using L-shaped indicators

I was introduced to this method for the first time more than 25 years ago, when two dowsers were making an energy map of my friend's apartment. The purpose of this investigation was to find optimum places for beds, tables and chairs and which places in the apartment should be avoided. As a result, a few small areas with negative energies were located. These areas could easily be avoided and my friends could spend more time in positive energy areas of the apartment. This is a good method to find artworks with positive energies as well.

I made my L-shaped rods myself just from scrap metal straight rods. See fig.7.B. I cut the rods and bent them to make L-shapes. I call them indicators. Some people make the indicators from wire coat hangers or use plastic rods instead of metal ones. Some people prefer to use metal or plastic handles to allow the indicators to swing more easily. See fig.7.A. You could make the handles using plastic pens. Remove the innards and caps of two pens, then put the indicator through the pen body. For me the indicators with handles are just too sensitive, moving all the time. So my indicators are just two pieces of metal rods, no handles. Elena prefers the indicators without handles, too. It's just a matter of personal preference. Choose what is comfortable for you and you will receive more reliable results.

I marked the left indicator with red tape and the right one with blue tape. Choose whatever color of tape you prefer.

Use the same indicators for right and left hands respectively. I found it will give you more reliable results in this case. I also bend the ends of the indicators to make them like small rings for safety reasons. See fig.7.B. You could also bend up the end of the left indicator and bend down the end of the right indicator. So you do not need to use the color tape to mark them.

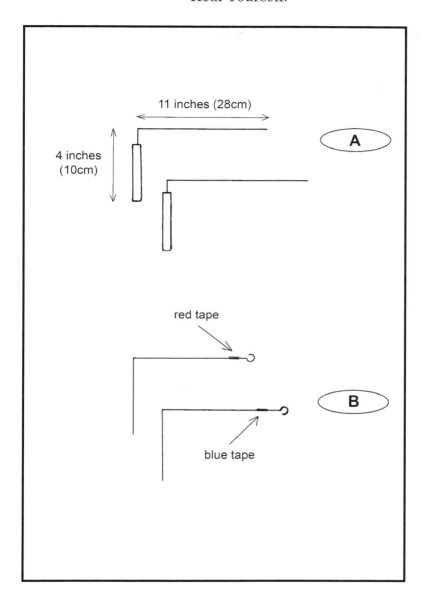

Fig.7. Dowsing method using L-shaped indicators

Ask your question to your Quantum DNA in a way that can be answered with just "Yes" or "No." Then, if the rods cross over one another making an X the answer is "Yes," but if they move away from each other the answer is "No". See fig.8.

As usual, you have to test it several times with questions for which you already know the answers. And when you have reliable answers try asking your main question.

Preparation

Use the following steps to prepare for the Dowsing method:

1. Go to a quiet room free of distractions like music or television.

2. For me, it works the best when I'm alone in the room, but you could do it with somebody else who is willing to do it with you.

3. Stand still, with your feet shoulder-width apart for a good balance. I place one indicator in each hand, with the short arm of the L held upright, and the long arm of the L pointing forward. I hold the indicators steady and straight in my hands, at arm's length from my body. See Fig.8.neutral. You could do it when you are standing or sitting. In the beginning, try sitting and standing and find what is most comfortable and reliable for you.

4. Let go of all worries and relax your body.

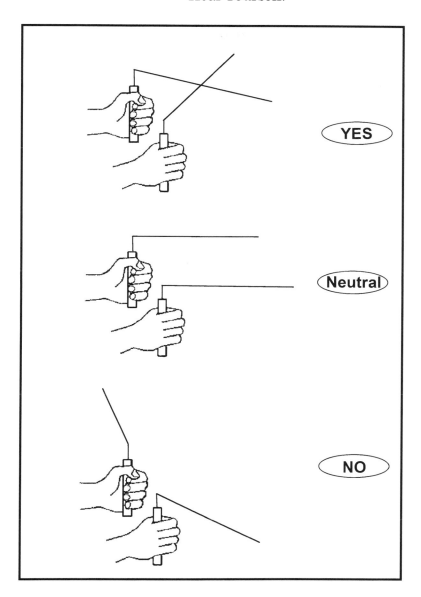

Fig.8. Dowsing method

5. Imagine that a golden-white light beam connects 3 points in your body: the heart, the heart chakra, and the crown chakra. See fig.2. This is my own addition to the standard method. If you are just starting to practice the dowsing method, you could skip this point, but I find that if I do it, I have more consistent results.

Perform the dowsing method

Perform the dowsing method using these steps:

1. Make a conscious attempt to communicate with your Quantum DNA. Say aloud, "I'm connected to my Quantum DNA."

2. To test that you have a connection, state aloud something that you know that is 100% true, for example, "My name is <your name>". In my case, I say "My name is Alexander".

   You are giving your subconscious mind, Quantum DNA a chance to speak to you in this way. Your subconscious mind, Quantum DNA knows what is true. When you make a true statement, the indicators begin to move and cross each other, usually within a few seconds. It means YES. See fig.8.

3. Continue testing the connection with your Quantum DNA. Make an untrue statement, for an example "my name is <somebody's name>". In my case I say "My name is Elena". As long as you choose a name that isn't yours, your subconscious mind will know that this statement is untrue. The indicators move away from each other, usually within a few seconds. It means NO. See fig.8.

4. Say "Neutral". The indicators rotate to the initial state. I do this in between any questions. I find

that it makes the results more reliable.

5. Repeat the true or false tests described in the previous steps several times in random order to make sure that you are getting reliable results before asking the main question for which you seek an answer.

6. State "I'm connected to my Quantum DNA". The indicators begin to rotate and cross each other, usually within a few seconds. It means that you are ready to communicate with your Quantum DNA.

7. Say "Neutral" to have the indicators move to the neutral state.

8. Now you are ready to ask your main question. Ask your question in a way that can be answered with just "Yes" or "No." Then if your indicators rotate and cross each other the answer is "Yes," but if the indicators rotate in opposite directions then the answer is "No." See fig.8.

Like most skills, your dowsing skill improves with practice.

We decided to have separate sets of indicators. So our personal energies will not influence the results.

Elena uses indicators very successfully. But I still prefer the Sway method, as it gives me more reliable results.

Do you want to try this method? I will give you an example how I do it and then you will try it on your own.

I initiate the connection as described above in the chapter. I always test the connection first, as described above.

I had the following conversation with my Quantum DNA.

Me: Dear Quantum DNA, is the print that I found emanating positive energy and good luck?
Quantum DNA: Yes.
Me: Thank you.

Now try to use the above example to find an artwork for your baby's room.

See pros and cons of using this method below.

Pros:

- You may sit or stand to use it
- Fast results

Cons:

- Not easy to use in public places without drawing attention to yourself
- For some people it's not possible to use it if they have any problems with their hands
- It's more difficult to learn, compared to the sway or pendulum methods. We are all different, so for you it may be easier to use this method than the others.

If for any reason you can't use the L-shaped indicators method, try the other methods listed in chapter 4. Try them until you find the one that is most suitable and reliable for you.

4.6 Shifting energy ball method

My wife Elena uses her own method. She calls it the Shifting Energy ball method. Elena told me that when she is feeling tired or lazy or if she needs a quick consultation, she mentally talks to her Quantum DNA. Often she does it while lying in a bed, sitting or walking. The body position doesn't matter, but it's important to be in an environment that is free of distractions. A strong intention, focus and a trust that information will come from a loving and benevolent Source is very vital. Being relaxed and open-minded is also very important.

Elena says that she senses a dense energy ball in her so-lar plexus (about 5" wide) as a YES response from her Quantum DNA. When the answer is NO, she senses the energy cloud in her back at the same level as the solar plexus. The neutral position is somewhere in the middle. See fig.9.

Sometimes she focuses in her mind on the similar test for connection that I do verbally. It goes something like this:

> *Elena: My dear Quantum DNA, can you hear me?*
> *Quantum DNA: Yes*
> *Elena: I love you*

After this often Elena senses chills along her spine and in limbs. It's a sign of a reliable connection and loving re-sponse from DNA. Then Elena asks her questions and gets answers in the form of the energy ball shifting for-ward or backward, as described earlier. Often she can sense answers even before finishing her question mental-ly.

She always ends session with gratitude:

> *Elena: Thank you so much my dear Quantum DNA. I love you.*

She feels the chilling sensation again as her body re-sponds with a message of love.

> *Elena: I'm disconnecting now.*
> *Quantum DNA: Yes*

Sometimes Elena skips the disconnection part. She falls asleep and stays in touch with her Quantum DNA until next session. That's OK, too.

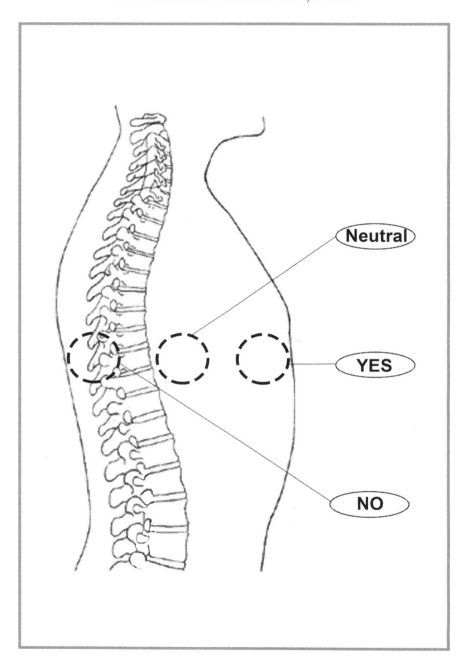

Fig.9. Shifting Energy ball method

See pros and cons of using this method below.

Pros:

- You may sit, lie down or stand to use it
- Could be used in public place without anybody noticing you
- Fast result

Cons:

- It can be more difficult to define sensations and learn it compare to sway, pendulum, or L-shaped indicators methods. However, we are all different so for you, it could be easier to use than other methods.

4.7 Conversations with my Quantum DNA

11th of January.

I initiated connection as described in chapter 4.3. I always test the connection first as the following:

> *Me: I'm connected to my Quantum DNA.*
> *Quantum DNA: Yes.*
> *Me: I'm Alexander.*
> *Quantum DNA: Yes.*
> *Me: Neutral.*
> *Me: I'm <somebody's name, for example Peter>.*
> *Quantum DNA: No.*

Sometimes I do this test several times to make sure that I am really connected. I always test the connection before any communications, so I'll be skipping the description of the test for the rest of the book.

I had the following conversation with my Quantum DNA.

> *Me: Dear Quantum DNA, would you heal me to be free from night pains in my chest in one day?*
> *Quantum DNA: No.*
> *Me: In 2 days?*
> *Quantum DNA: Yes.*

12th of January.

At night, I was woken up by pains again. I drank some herbal tea, then used my healing electric pulse device on the 7 acupuncture points. Sometime later the pain decreased and I went to sleep.

13th of January.

I had a good effective sleep (remember that on 11th of January the Quantum DNA responded, that my pain would be healed in 2 days), and woke up with a healthy and happy face. I had a nice run even though the temperature outside was -18°C.

I find that I am getting a connection to my Quantum DNA faster and faster every day.

14th of January.

My wife Elena found an interesting video about water and asked me to watch it. This reminded me that I have a device that I built myself a long time ago. This electrical device makes Living Water that is alkaline and has powerful healing properties. I decided to ask the Quantum DNA about the Living Water and about some other things.

I initiated connection and tested it as described in chapter 4.3 and started the following conversation.

> *Me: Is the Living Water good for healing me now?*
> *Quantum DNA: Yes.*
> *Me: Are the Sea buckthorn berries good for healing me now?*
> *Quantum DNA: Yes.*
> *Me: Are the frozen green beans from our garden good for healing me now?*
> *Quantum DNA: Yes.*

21st of January

I initiated connection and tested it as described in chapter 4.3 and started the following conversation.

> *Me: Are black currants with honey good for my breakfast right now?*
> *Quantum DNA: No.*
> *Me: Are raspberries with honey good for my breakfast right now?*
> *Quantum DNA: No.*
> *Me: Are oranges good for my breakfast right now?*
> *Quantum DNA: No.*

Me: Are sea buckthorn berries good for my breakfast right now?
Quantum DNA: Yes.

I have asked about the sea buckthorn berries before, but I decided to ask again in case something had changed.

5th of February.

I initiated the connection and tested it as described in chapter 4.3 and started the following conversation.

Me: Is the EFT calming technique one of the main turning points to heal my night pains right now?
Quantum DNA: Yes.
Me: Is a honey massage one of the main turning points to heal my night pains right now?
Quantum DNA: No.
Me: Is a regular massage one of the main turning points to heal my night pains right now?
Quantum DNA: No.
Me: Are honey and regular massages helpful as an addition but not as a main turning point to heal my night pains right now?
Quantum DNA: Yes.

Did you notice how important it is to have a carefully crafted question to get an answer you are looking for? Based on the previous conversation, I used EFT (Energy Tapping Technique) for a quick energy boost. Being in a good energetic shape is very important, especially if you find yourself in health challenging situation.

For breakfast I had fermented beans with sour cream. I excluded black currant, oranges, raspberries and sea buckthorn berries. I had 7 components herbal tea with valerian roots several times during the day. At supper I had some cheese and sour cream and herbal tea with valerian roots. I had used a calming EFT before sleep. The result was a nice sleep with no waking during night.

6th of February.

At breakfast I had a cottage cheese with bananas. I had herbal tea with valerian roots several times during the day to heal myself. At lunch I had some fermented beans with sour cream. At supper I had steamed salmon with slightly boiled sprouted mung beans, raw sunflower seeds and tea with valerian roots. I had a calming EFT before sleep. I had a nice sleep again.

10th of February.

It was a fasting day and I had just herbal tea but without valerian roots. At night I was awakened by pains in the chest again. I treated the 7 acupuncture points using my special device for half an hour. After that, I was able to go to sleep.

11th of February.

During my morning run in the park I stopped by the river and spoke to my Quantum DNA.

I initiated the connection and tested it as described in chapter 4.3 and started the following conversation.

> *Me: Can you do all my requests, which I have asked before in comfortable pace?*
> *Quantum DNA: Yes.*

In the evening I had 2 cups of herbal tea with valerian root. That night, I woke with chest pains again. I treated the acupuncture points using my special device for half an hour and then went to sleep.

12th of February.

Today I had a sore throat (tonsillitis). I started healing myself with herbal rinses and herbal tea, without medications. I decided to ask my Quantum DNA to help me.

I initiated connection and tested it as described in chapter 4.3 and started the following conversation.

> *Me: Can you heal my throat in 24 hours?*
> *Quantum DNA: No.*
> *Me: Can you heal my throat in 2 days?*
> *Quantum DNA: No.*
> *Me: Can you heal my throat in 4 days?*
> *Quantum DNA: Yes.*

13th of February.

I was healing my throat with herbal tea and herbal rinses. I also had some consultations with my Quantum DNA.

I initiated connection and tested it as described in chapter 4.3 and started the following conversation.

> *Me: Can I have a shower today?*
> *Quantum DNA: No.*
> *Me: Can I have a bath today?*
> *Quantum DNA: No.*

14th of February.

I was healing my throat with herbal tea and herbal rinses. I contacted with my Quantum DNA again.

I initiated connection and tested it as described in chapter 4.3 and started the following conversation.

> *Me: Can I have a shower today?*
> *Quantum DNA: No.*
> *Me: Can I have a bath today?*
> *Quantum DNA: No.*

15th of February.

I was healing my throat with herbal tea and herbal rinses. I had the same questions as yesterday to my Quantum

DNA and got the same answers.

16th of February.

My throat felt completely healed by the end of day. I had just one question to my Quantum DNA.

Me: Can I have a shower today?
Quantum DNA: Yes.

I was very happy. I slept well all night without any pain in the chest.

For most of the days in February I was doing the following things:

- Working to improve our www.LightFromArt.com website. It was a difficult time, because art is the first thing that suffers in a recession. I was worried about it.

- Sending the Good Luck energy to others first.

- Last thing that I was doing if I had some time is to love myself, and for sure it wasn't enough.

5. The message from Gosha: Love yourself first or die

The more often I practiced connecting to my Quantum DNA, the faster I was able to connect. I always tested the connections as described earlier.

During one session I got an unexpected message: our family angel, our budgie, Gosha, was dying. I didn't believe it, but one week later, on February 20th at 2 p.m., he suddenly died peacefully. We were in shock.

Elena saw Gosha's aura sitting on his favorite branch at night. I heard his voice several times, as if he was still at home. We wished him to be reincarnated and come back to us.

In one of my meditations I asked the question:

"Why Did Gosha die?"

Suddenly I realized that he died to give me a strong message that I have to love myself first and care about myself more, otherwise I'll die.

Now I realized that I was in pain for more than 8 months, because I didn't do this. Any powerful healing method will fail if I do not love myself first. So I have to change my bad habits now and then I can bring more love to others.

I took Gosha's strong message to heart. I started to develop a new habit of loving myself first, then sharing my love with others. It sounds easy, but in reality it is a very difficult task, at least it was for me. When you are doing some exciting projects or you are very busy, it is easy to ignore your own needs. Sound familiar? I remembered the preparation for our overseas trip and the sleepless night just before we left. I remembered preparing for important exams.

So I decided to work hard to develop new habits. I also needed to improve my health as the base for the rest of the changes that I needed to make in my life. I felt that I needed some direction.

So I decided to consult with my Quantum DNA about the food I ate.

I initiated connection and tested it as described in chapter 4.3 and started the following conversation.

Me: Is a millet porridge good for me to eat now?
Quantum DNA: Yes.

I also asked about the following foods and got the answer YES from my Quantum DNA: nori, kelp, vermicelli brown rice, brown rice, white rice, popped rice, quinoa, Alaskan Pollack, bus fish, soul fish, broccoli, celery, carrots, carrot juice, olives, cucumbers, pears, peaches, blackberries, sunflower seed, almonds, walnuts, filbert, coconuts, sweet grapes, watermelon, cantaloupe, sweet apples, bananas, oranges, avocados, cauliflower, raisins, prunes, beets, red pepper, strawberries, grape oil, olive oil, rye bread, cabbage, kefir from 3.5% milk, cheese, feta, bakers cheese.

Me: Is a buckwheat porridge good for me to eat now?
Quantum DNA: No.

I also asked about the following foods and got the answer NO from my Quantum DNA: butter, meat, borodinskii bread, sour cream, oatmeal, smoked sprats, smoked sturgeon fish, maple walnut ice-cream, potatoes chips, chocolate, coffee, black tea, eggs, salmon, tilapia, cod, chicken, goose, turkey, raspberries, lemons, milk, cream, cottage cheese, tomato juice, black pepper, vinegar, ketchup, garlic, brandy.

I included this list of foods in the Appendix in this book. You can use that list to ask your Quantum DNA about the foods that are best for you and your family.

I also asked about the following.

> *Me: Are morning and evening runs helpful for me to heal faster?*
> *Quantum DNA: Yes.*
> *Me: Are Donna Eden's 5 minute energy exercises helpful for me to heal faster?*
> *Quantum DNA: Yes.*
> *Me: Is honey massage helpful for me to heal faster?*
> *Quantum DNA: Yes.*

To build a healthy foundation I decided to do the following things every day:

In the morning:

- Positive affirmations (see chapter 2)
- 2-3 km run
- Donna Eden's 5 minute energy exercises [1]
- Drink a healing tea made with 7 herbs

During the day:

- After 45 minutes of work on the computer, take a break of at least 15 minutes. Do something active.

In the evening:

- 2-3 km run
- Honey massage (10 days complete set)
- Go sleep on time. It doesn't matter what time as

long as it is the same time every night.

- Always get enough sleep.

To make my working day more pleasant and productive I decluttered my home office. I also put a special metaphysical energy art painting "Opening to Love" [8] on the wall just in front of my desk. Elena created it to bring a good luck and love energy to the room. Near the front door I had a "Prosperity" art print [9] that Elena created to bring good luck and prosperity. Before the art print was just pinned to the wall, but now I stretched the canvas of the print on a frame and it looks fantastic. Beside me I placed a canvas print from my photograph "Roses for Love" [10], which I created to bring love and good luck. I framed it, too, just for this occasion. So I have surrounded myself with Love, Good Luck and beautiful inspiring art.

I also cleaned up my 2 white boards. I started to use one of them just for items on how to improve my health and for reminders how to love myself first. My office looks so great now and I have more productive days. Now I have more time to love myself too. The results are amazing since I established my new habits.

From 24th of February until 6th of March.

I got a honey massage every day, except March 1st. So I got 7 massages. For 8 days I slept well without any pains at night and felt great the next day.

7th and 8th of March.

I was very busy with preparations for International Women's day and didn't love myself enough. I didn't have a honey massage either.

9th of March.

Very early in the morning I had some chest pains again. It was a very powerful reminder, so on the evening on 9th of March I had the 8th healing honey massage and slept well without any pains.

From 10th to 13th of March.

I had a honey massage every day. Each night I slept well without any pains and I felt stronger every day.

24th of March at 12.30 am.

After 2 weeks without any pain in my chest I got strong pain in the heart chakra. So I decided to talk to my Quantum DNA.

I initiated connection and tested it as described in chapter 4.3 and started the following conversation.

> *Me: Did I have the pain because of the shift to new energies again?*
> *Quantum DNA: Yes.*
> *Me: Dear Quantum DNA could you accept new energy now and in the future only at a comfortable pace, so I'll not feel pain?*
> *Quantum DNA: Yes.*
> *Me: Dear Quantum DNA, could you clean my body of any old energies?*
> *Quantum DNA: Yes.*

I felt more comfortable just after the conversation, with some traces of the pain, but not enough to disturb my sleep.

For the next 4 days I felt very good and free from any pain in my chakras.

27th of March.

I felt some pain in the bump on my eyelid. I have had this bump for years without any problems. Some time ago, I visited an eye doctor to check on it. He told me that it was nothing to worry about and I could easily live with it. It could be removed by surgery, but I didn't want to do that at this point.

28th of March.

My left eyelid was swollen and painful. It has swollen to 5 times the size of the bump. I decided to ask my Quantum DNA for help.

I initiated connection and tested it as described at chapter 4.3 and started the following conversation.

> *Me: Dear Quantum DNA, could you completely heal my eyelid today?*
> *Quantum DNA: No.*
> *Me: Can you completely heal my eyelid tomorrow?*
> *Quantum DNA: Yes.*
> *Me: Will an application of a propolis tincture to the eye lid be useful to heal it?*
> *Quantum DNA: Yes.*

I applied it at 8.30 am. By the afternoon, the swollen area had decreased to half its size.

The pain had decreased too, but not completely. I decided to apply the propolis tincture again at 1.25 pm.

Then I talked to my Quantum DNA again.

I initiated connection and tested it as described in chapter 4.3 and started the following conversation.

> *Me: Can you completely remove the bump from my eye lid?*
> *Quantum DNA: Yes.*
> *Me: Can you do it by tomorrow?*
> *Quantum DNA: No.*
> *Me: Can you do it in one week?*
> *Quantum DNA: No.*
> *Me: Can you do it in two weeks?*
> *Quantum DNA: No.*
> *Me: Can you do it in one month?*

Quantum DNA: Yes.
Me: Please do.
Me: Can you heal any bad things in my body even if I don't know about them yet?
Quantum DNA: Yes.
Me: Please do.

29th of March.

The swollen area on my eyelid disappeared and I was free from all the pain. But the bump on my eyelid looked bigger than usual, and I felt uncomfortable. So I decided to check up with Quantum DNA again.

I initiated connection and tested it as described in chapter 4.3 and started the following conversation.

Me: Is the bump on my eye lid bigger than usual because I asked you to remove it and you are doing it right now?
Quantum DNA: Yes.
Me: Please do, but heal the bump area first for now.
Quantum DNA: Yes.
Me: Can you do it today?
Quantum DNA: No.
Me: Can you do it tomorrow?
Quantum DNA: Yes.
Me: Please do.

30th of March.

The bump was healed.

3rd of April.

In the middle of the day I felt some small uncomfortable pain in the chest. So I asked my Quantum DNA for help.

I initiated connection and tested it as described in chapter 4.3 and started the following conversation.

Me: Is the pain related to the shifting of new energies?

> *Quantum DNA: Yes.*
> *Me: Can you heal it today?*
> *Quantum DNA: Yes.*
> *Me: Please do. You have my permanent permission to do all necessary adjustments to new energies but only at a pace that is comfortable for me. Could you do it for me?*
> *Quantum DNA: Yes.*
> *Me: Please do.*

I felt good after my conversation with my Quantum DNA.

After that I had a good night's sleep. I felt very good the next day. That day I continued to ask questions about food that was good for me:

I initiated connection and tested it as described in chapter 4.3 and started the following conversation.

> *Me: Is salmon good for me to eat?*
> *Quantum DNA: No.*

I asked this question before, but I was hoping that something changed and answer would be YES, but again the answer was NO.

I also asked about the following foods and my Quantum DNA answered YES: three kinds of fish: bass, sole, Alaskan Pollock, and cottage cheese.

I had some strain in my left eye when reading books that day. So I made the following request to my Quantum DNA. I initiated connection and tested it as described in chapter 4.3 and started the following conversation.

> *Me: Could you heal my eyes?*
> *Quantum DNA: Yes.*
> *Me: Could you heal my eyes today?*
> *Quantum DNA: No.*
> *Me: Could you heal my eyes tomorrow?*
> *Quantum DNA: Yes.*
> *Me: Please do.*

4th of April.

I noticed that I didn't have strain in my eyes after asking my Quantum DNA to heal it yesterday.

5th of April.

Our Christmas cactus is flowering today! I photographed it and put it on my Facebook page and sent my love to my friends.

I noticed that I sent my love to thousands of my friends, but I forgot to love myself again. I didn't do my morning energy exercises either.

Continue talking to my Quantum DNA.

I initiated connection and tested it as described in chapter 4.3 and started the following conversation.

> *Me: Is it good for me to drink beer?*
> *Quantum DNA: No.*
> *Me: Just a little bit?*
> *Quantum DNA: No.*
> *Me: Is it good for me to drink red wine?*
> *Quantum DNA: No.*
> *Me: Just a little bit?*
> *Quantum DNA: No.*
> *Me: Is it good for me to eat ice cream?*
> *Quantum DNA: No.*

Finally in the evening I found some time to do energy exercises (instead of first thing in the morning).

6th of April.

I had a good night's sleep. I was so happy. Thank you Quantum DNA! I noticed some small pain in the right side of my chest for few seconds and then again half an hour later.

I initiated connection and tested it as described in chapter 4.3 and started the following conversation.

Me: Could you heal my pain now?
Quantum DNA: Yes.
Me: Please do.

It was done at once! Miracle! I felt so good. I was so grateful.

Me: Thank you spirit! Could you heal anything in my body that I even don't know about yet?
Quantum DNA: Yes.
Me: Could you heal it by tomorrow morning?
Quantum DNA: Yes.
Me: Please do.

I like to eat ice cream, but my Quantum DNA answered NO. I decided to ask it again. Perhaps something had changed?

Me: Is it good for me to eat ice cream now?
Quantum DNA: No.
Me: Is it good for me to eat a maple walnut ice cream now?
Quantum DNA: No.
Me: Is it good for me to eat a goat milk organic ice cream?
Quantum DNA: Yes.

This was good news for me!

Most days I use my new habits of eating food that is good for my health. I felt better and better every day.

6. At last I feel cured

Finally, I am healthy again! On April 7th, I awoke after a good night's sleep feeling very happy! I looked in the mirror. WOW: my eyes emanate light, my cheeks are rounded, and I look very healthy. I am back to my normal weight. It doesn't matter what I eat, my weight is very stable. Thank you, Quantum DNA! Finally, I feel completely cured after almost a year!

I went to my computer to send Light and Love to my Facebook friends without first making positive affirmations and doing my energy exercises. I caught myself on it. "Oh, boy, my old habits are still trying to win, but I'm alert and watching now!" I asked my wife to join me.

> *Me: Elena! Let's do affirmations and energy exercises together.*
> *Elena: I am very busy in the garden. I have to finish pruning today.*
> *Me: Gosha sacrificed his life to send us a message that we have to love ourselves first to be able to send more light to other people. Do you want our new baby budgie, Joy, to send the same message again?*
> *Elena: No, but I am busy...*
> *Me: Let's at least do affirmations, then. It only takes*

a minute.
Elena: OK.

Hooray... We did it.

Later in the day...

Me: It's already 2.30 pm and we haven't had lunch yet. Let's do it now.
Elena: I don't want to...

Elena was busy. So I decided I'd like to love myself and have lunch at the same time.

One hour later:

Elena: I was thinking about your words. Let's have lunch and do the energy exercises now.
Me: Great! I had my lunch already. But I'll do energy exercises with pleasure.

And so we did. I felt so refreshed, as always after energy exercises.

And I went with Joy (our budgie) to write about it.

Joy was sitting on my shoulder, inspiring me.

Later, I got a phone call from a gallery. The gallery was closing up and our business relationship was coming to an end. I was very surprised about my reaction to the news. If I had received the same news a few months ago, I would have grieved and been full of anxiety. Instead, I was thankful for the 20 years of good cooperation I had with the gallery. I sincerely wished good luck to the owner. Somehow I felt that it was happening for my highest good and that a new and better source of income would come in the future. It seems my request to my Quantum DNA to help me let go of fear is working well!

I'm cured, but to stay healthy and to bring more LIGHT to the people I have to love myself first.

6.1 Three easy steps for Healing, Good Luck, Love, Joy and much more...

Three healing steps that I used are the following:

1. Love yourself first
2. Connect to your Quantum DNA
3. Ask your Quantum DNA to heal you in a comfortable pace. Be open and trust the process. Be grateful for the outcome.

*   *   *

I have consulted with my Spiritual DNA to get advice in many different aspects of my life, including my books, healing art, joy... Discover more examples at

http://lightfromart.com/gifts.

I always ask my Spiritual DNA to give me what I ask in a comfortable pace. I found that it's a very important to remember to ask about it.

I continue to communicate to my Quantum DNA and Higher Self to enhance my life and stay healthy and happy.

Conclusions

I hope this book has given you an inspiration to use the power within you, your Quantum DNA and Higher Self to have a happy, joyful and prosperous life.

My healing is within me. Instead of fighting against the nature of the universe in order to heal, I asked my Quantum DNA to heal me.

I became ill because I was so caught up in pursuing goals, achieving, and helping others. I considered myself last.

Now, unconditional self-love increases my energy. The external world mirrors what is within me. I love myself, so there is more love around me too. I give more to others than before.

Any positivity you bring to yourself, you are bringing to all the people around you. Start to love yourself, and this love will help you and everybody else, because we are all connected - we are ONE.

Sending you LIGHT and LOVE☺.

Dr. Alexander Khomoutov

My confessions to you

Now I am cured and feel so good. I sleep well. I enjoy some foods that I couldn't eat before. My weight is very stable and optimal for me. I have had the most joyful year of my life. However, from time to time I catch myself forgetting to love myself first. For example, today I caught myself sending a birthday gift video "Meditation for a good healing sleep" [7] to my three Facebook friends. I was doing it before my positive affirmations and energy exercises. I have to do those exercises before anything else. So, I turned my computer off, did all of my exercises, and then went back to congratulate my Facebook friends.

From time to time, when I was working on some exciting project, including this book, I would catch myself working without any breaks for several hours or working late into the night. So I stopped doing it, reminded myself to love myself first. Love is most powerful healer for me and for all of us. If you love yourself first, then you can spread more love and peace around the world.

Alexander

Questions and Answers

After the release of my first edition of "How to Heal Yourself", I received questions from readers. The following are some of the answers that have resulted from those conversations.

Q: I noticed that you "cured" your problem with your DNA system but you did not find a root cause for it.

A: The root of the problem was that I asked my Quantum DNA to uplift my energy frequency but I did not ask to do it at a comfortable pace. My body was not ready for those rapid changes. Another reason was a presence of old energies, that didn't serve me anymore. As a result, I had unbalanced energies and many pains. All of the above were amplified by <<< not loving myself enough>>>. Now I always ask my Quantum DNA to do all my requests at a comfortable pace. From time to time I ask my Quantum DNA to remove my old energies.

Q: It is good for people to try this method of looking at their health, alongside medical advice. They are not mutually exclusive.

A: Yes, I agree with you. The information received from the book should not in any way be used as a substitute for

advice from a medical advisor or other licensed professionals.

Q: I think the shopping lists of your meals is not neces-
sary. It would have been better to show some healthy eating meals and recipes in an appendix at the end of the
book.

A: When I was healing myself I needed to know which
foods were supporting my efforts and which were not. So I
used the table to keep track of foods. I retested it from
time to time because some foods that were bad for me
when I was in the beginning of the healing became good
for me when I was cured. So the tables are not for advice
but for tracking the changes in food compatibility. I added
an example of how I use the tables in the beginning of
Appendix. I have also divided the table into several
smaller tables for ease of use. Your question inspired me
to do so. Thank you.

Q: I cannot do the swaying method, because of spinal
problems. Could ordinary dowsing work for your Quantum DNA system?

A: Yes, the ordinary dowsing works, too. I have used the
ordinary dowsing method for more than 45 years. Any
Applied Kinesiology methods will work to communicate
with your Quantum DNA. We are all unique, so the
methods that will work best for us might be different. In
the first edition, I focused on the Sway method because it
worked best for me.

Your question inspired me to add several chapters with
other methods I personally have used. Thank you.

Q: Hi Alexander!! I have been working on connecting with
my Quantum DNA and it is a journey just like you
shared. My body decided that it was not ready for a dental
surgery. So it got this cold cough issue. Pills were not
helping. I talked to my body and used a surprise treat-

ment that I have been told by others and it didn't work. I think it's a reinforcement that I also need to be careful of sharing what works with me with others. Since throwing the negative on it does not allow it to keep working for me as well. I just wanted to say I am far from getting on your level of having this work but I am over the top excited about how far I have come. This has helped me stop the crazy coughing I was doing yesterday. Is there some focus you use so the demons of others do not interfere with your healing??? Please have an awesome day!! Thank you so very much!!

A: I hope to bring as much healing light as I can through social networking and in my books. I share everything as it is because those who are ready will get it. If they are not ready, they are free not to read it.

If you already shared your ideas with your friends who are not ready to understand it now and they responded negatively, then send love and light to all of them now.

But most importantly, you have to believe in yourself. At the moment you believe in yourself you will succeed at the same level as me or higher. Send your love and light to yourself!

Sending you healing light and good luck energy.

Q (continuation of the previous conversation): Thank you Alexander for first being open to helping me see things in a better perspective. I had only shared my supplement and product ideas and that too since I must not be in a good place was met with anger and lecturing. This seems to of curtail my believing in myself. I greatly appreciate you sharing this with me. I am sending you healing light and love back. Thank you so very much and I hope you feel some magic today!

A: You are welcome. Sending more healing light your way.

Q: Did you heal somebody else using Quantum DNA? Could you tell me how you have done it step by step?

A: On 22d of March, Elena had a strong headache at night and as a result she had a bad sleep. She did not want to get up in the morning because of the strong headache. I offered to heal her using the Quantum DNA method. I got her permission and connected to my Quantum DNA first. I spoke loud enough so that Elena could listen to the whole session.

> Me: Am I connected to my Quantum DNA.
> Quantum DNA: Yes.
> Me: I'm Alexander.
> Quantum DNA: Yes.
> Me: Neutral.
> Me: I'm Elena.
> Quantum DNA: No.

I repeated the above test one more time to make sure that I was really connected.

> Me: Dear Quantum DNA, connect to Elena's Quantum DNA. Do I have a connection?
> Elena's Quantum DNA: Yes.
> Me speaking to Elena's DNA: Please cure the root cause of the headache. Heal any diseases Elena has now, even those that she isn't aware of. Use a youth template to create all new cells now and in the future. Elena's skin is getting younger and younger every day.
> Elena's Quantum DNA: Yes.
> Me speaking to Elena's DNA: Thank you Quantum DNA, for connection and help.
> Elena's Quantum DNA: Yes.
> Me: I'm disconnected from Elena's Quantum DNA now.
> Elena's Quantum DNA: Yes

Then I tested that I was really disconnected from Elena's Quantum DNA.

Me: I am Elena.
My Quantum DNA: No.
Me: I am Alexander.
My Quantum DNA: Yes.
Elena: Thank you, I feel so good now.
Me: You should wake me up next time you have a headache at night and I will heal you.
Elena: I will!

The healing was done instantly.

I also tried to help to couple of my friends. They gave me permission to do it, but they didn't believe that it was possible. Do you know what was happened? You are right. It didn't work. When I was writing about it in this book, I connected to my Quantum DNA and discovered that my friends' disbelief blocked the healing in both cases.

Q: Could you give us new examples of using Quantum DNA to heal yourself?

A: On 23th of December I was shopping for tasty food and flowers for Elena. I went to a small store packed with a lot of delicious things that Elena loves. I just entered the store and was trying to get a shopping basket using my left hand but suddenly I saw an owner of the store close to me. At this exact second my finger went between the metal door and door frame. The rest probably you already know. Suddenly I felt a huge pain in my finger before I had even had a chance to say hello. At this moment I forgot that I could use a powerful healing connection with my Quantum DNA. In shock, I put my painful, bleeding finger in my mouth. The store owner's wife recommended that I wash finger and she gave me a bottle of a hydrogen peroxide and a bandage. I washed my finger and applied the bandage. Suddenly, I saw myself in the mirror and didn't recognize myself. My face was so pale and the pain was so huge, that I was frightened. Then I got the idea to connect to my Quantum DNA and ask to cure my finger. I initiated the connection, tested it as described in chapter 4.3 and started the following conversation.

Me: Dear Quantum DNA please instantly heal my finger.
Quantum DNA: Yes.
Me: Thank you.

Just in few seconds after that the pain was diminished so dramatically, that I felt good enough to continue shopping. I found everything what Elena wanted from this store and was relaxed and smiling when I was leaving the store. I felt good enough to continue my shopping and visited several stores after this. When I got home Elena didn't sense what had happened. But at the end of the day she asked me: "Did anything unusual happen today? And I told her my story.

The next day I was typing this book using this finger without noticeable pain. Just some sensations that something happened with my finger, a little bit deformed nail, a bruise under my nail and scratches around the nail.

A few days later I had another healing case. I felt some small pains in the heart area of my chest in the morning. I started to use old ways first: meditation, a breathing technique, and a special herbal tea. I didn't have any improvements in my condition by the end of the day. Suddenly I realized that I forgot about the most powerful healing method using my Quantum DNA. So I initiated connection and tested it as described in chapter 4.3 and started the following conversation.

Me: Dear Quantum DNA please instantly heal the root of the pain in my chest.
Quantum DNA: Yes.
Me: Thank you.

Just in few seconds after that the pain was diminished dramatically. Elena and I went out for an hour of amazing skiing in the local fields.

Do you know how powerful you are? I have to confess - I forget sometimes how powerful I am and use old ways first. Today, as I was cycling on the road, a wasp stung my leg. First I tried to find a plantain plant near the road to put on it, but I couldn't find one. Then I decided to use my power. I connected to my Quantum DNA and set it for curing. A minute later the pain almost gone and I continued cycling and enjoying the day.

It reminds me that I should use both traditional and Quantum DNA methods from the start!

I should create a new habit to do it at same time. When I was writing about it, I got an idea to have a special Quantum DNA session and ask to help me to create this habit for me. I stopped writing the book and just did the following:

> *Me: Dear Quantum DNA please create a new habit for me to start using Quantum DNA method at the same time as traditional healing methods.*
> *Quantum DNA: Yes.*
> *Me: Thank you.*

Recently I decided to be connected to my Quantum DNA 24/7. This way I can directly ask my Quantum DNA anything without initiating the conversation.

I initiated connection and tested it as described in chapter 4.3 and started the following special conversation.

> *Me: Dear Quantum DNA please connect me to my Quantum DNA 24/7. As I am constantly connected, please heal anything in my body, even if I haven't noticed it yet. Use the youth template to create my new cells and rejuvenate my body, so I could live longer with good health and joy.*
> *Quantum DNA: Yes.*

Me: Thank you.

I do not need to connect any more. I just ask what I want to achieve at this point. For now, I still test that I'm connected first and then ask what I need. But in the future if I find that I'm always connected, I will drop the testing of the connection with my Quantum DNA too.

Q: In your book you wrote about your wife's experience in relocating ants using Quantum DNA communications. Did you relocate ants yourself too?

A: Yes. I was planning to put some caulking in the gap between the driveway and the garage floor this year. I found that ants had made a nest in the gap. I connected to my Quantum DNA and asked the ants to relocate in 24 hours. 2 days later I checked the gap and I did not find the ants. Do you think that it's just a coincidence? But this is my second case of relocating ants this year.

Maybe you think that I'm very special. But my wife Elena has done it 2 times and our friend has done it too. In our friend's case, ants were in the basement. She tried traditional methods and traps. Nothing worked until she tried to talk to the ants. So try it! The results will speak for themselves. And you will believe even more how powerful you are.

Q: Could you give us an example of using Quantum DNA to heal pets?

A: We have a budgie named Joy. Usually budgies lay 4 or 5 eggs and then stop, but she was laying one egg every second day for more than 2 months and she was very exhausted. We tried all the solutions what we found but none of them worked. After Joy has laid 32 eggs, I decided to help her to stop by using the Quantum DNA method.

I connected to my Quantum DNA and tested a connection using the same procedure as in my previous examples and then I had the following conversation.

Me: Dear Quantum DNA, connect to Joy's Quantum DNA. Do I have a connection?
Joy's Quantum DNA: Yes.
Me speaking to Joy's DNA: Joy is free of eggs.
Joy's Quantum DNA: Yes.
Me speaking to Joy's DNA: Thank you Quantum DNA, for connection and help.
Joy's Quantum DNA: Yes.
Me: I'm disconnected from Joy's Quantum DNA now.
Joy's Quantum DNA: Yes

Then I tested that I was really disconnected from Joy's Quantum DNA as I did at previous examples.

Joy laid one egg the next day after the DNA session and then she stopped laying eggs.

Since then, I have used Quantum DNA sessions not only for healing Joy but for training her. The results have been great. Discover more about it in my next book, coming soon. Visit http://lightfromart.com/Dr-AK-books for details.

Thank you for all your questions. Please feel welcome to ask more.

Appendix: Food list for the Quantum DNA test for you and your family

You are unique, so it makes sense that your diet— the foods that heal you and that you should avoid —is also unique. Use the following lists to keep track as you test the foods that are good for you and your family members.

I usually initiate a connection with my Quantum DNA as described in chapter 4.3 of the book and start the following conversation.

> *Me: Is a mint tea good for me?*
> *Quantum DNA: Yes.*

Do a similar test for the rest of items. If you are planning to test many of them, then recheck your connection to your Quantum DNA periodically. Use a question for which you know the correct answer, for example your name and somebody else's name. If you get the right response, then continue your session. Sometime if you try to write down all answers you could lose the connection.

For a free download of these tables in pdf format, go to: www.LightFromArt.com/gifts .

Print it and use it. See below an example of using the table for you and 4 members of your family.

#	Name	You	1	2	3	4
1.	Herbal chamomile tea	+	-	-	-	-
2.	Black tea	-	+	-	+	-
3.	Coffee	-	-	+	+	+

Put plus symbols for items with positive Quantum DNA responses and minus symbols for items with negative responses.

I would suggest to test one table at the time. Put results in the table. Check out that you are still connected to your Quantum DNA and then test another table. Otherwise, reconnect to your Quantum DNA first as described in chapter 4.3 and then continue your food testing.

How often should you recheck your food list? You are unique so the answer will be different for each person. Connect to your Quantum DNA and ask the following question:

Me: Dear Quantum DNA! Are all my food test results still valid?
Quantum DNA: Yes.

If the answer is Yes then your food test results are still valid. If the answer is No then retest all lists. See example below.

Me: Are the diary list test results still valid?
Quantum DNA: Yes.
Me: Are the drinks list test results still valid?
Quantum DNA: No.

Continue asking similar questions for the rest of the lists to find all tables that you should recheck and retest all items on those ones.

The lists below are just the basic initial ones to start with. You are unique so is your food compatibility. If you will not find something on the list then add it at the bottom of the tables or at table 14 and 15, which I created just for you.

The tables are basic ones just to start with. If you do not eat some foods, cross them out in the tables and never test them.

Dr. Alexander Khomoutov, Ph.D.

When I was ill, I tested all foods that I usually eat to find out what foods to avoid. However, after I completely cured I only retest food that I felt intuitively I would have to.

Table 1. Fresh Vegetables

#	Name	You	1	2	3	4
1.	Asparagus					
2.	Beets					
3.	Broccoli					
4.	Cabbage					
5.	Carrots					
6.	Cauliflower					
7.	Celery					
8.	Corn					
9.	Cucumbers					
10.	Lettuce					
11.	Mushrooms					
12.	Onions					
13.	Peppers					
14.	Potatoes					
15.	Spinach					
16.	Squash					
17.	Tomatoes					
18.	Zucchini					

Table 2. Fresh fruits

#	Name	You	1	2	3	4
1.	Apples					
2.	Avocados					
3.	Bananas					
4.	Blueberries					
5.	Cherries					
6.	Grapefruit					
7.	Grapes					
8.	Lemons					
9.	Limes					
10.	Melon					
11.	Nectarines					
12.	Oranges					
13.	Peaches					
14.	Pears					
15.	Plums					
16.	Raspberries					
17.	Strawberries					

Table 3. Dairy

#	Name	You	1	2	3	4
1.	Butter					
2.	Goat milk					
3.	Half & Half Cream					
4.	Kefir					
5.	Milk					
6.	Organic Butter					
7.	Organic Milk					
8.	Organic Sour Cream					
9.	Sour Cream					
10.	Whipped cream					
11.	Yogurt					
Add your other favorite items below						
12.						
13.						
14.						
15.						
16.						

Table 4. Cheese

#	Name	You	1	2	3	4
1.	Blue cheese	.				
2.	Cheddar					
3.	Coconut cheese					
4.	Cottage cheese					
5.	Cream cheese					
6.	Feta					
7.	Goat cheese					
8.	Mozzarella					
9.	Parmesan					
10.	Provolone					
11.	Ricotta					
12.	Sandwich slices					
13.	Swiss					
Add your other favorite items below						
14.						
15.						
16.						

Table 5. Meat

#	Name	You	1	2	3	4
1.	Bacon					
2.	Beef					
3.	Chicken					
4.	Ground beef					
5.	Ham					
6.	Hot dogs					
7.	Lunchmeat					
8.	Pork					
9.	Sausage					
10.	Turkey					
Add your other favorite items below						
11.						
12.						
13.						
14.						
15.						
16.						

Table 6. Seafood

#	Name	You	1	2	3	4
1.	Bass					
2.	Catfish					
3.	Cod					
4.	Crab					
5.	Haddock					
6.	Lobster					
7.	Mussels					
8.	Oysters					
9.	Pollock					
10.	Salmon					
11.	Shrimp					
12.	Sole					
13.	Tilapia					
14.	Tuna					
Add your other favorite items below						
15.						
16.						

Table 7. Nuts and seeds

#	Name	You	1	2	3	4
1.	Almonds					
2.	Brazil Nuts					
3.	Cashews					
4.	Hazelnuts					
5.	Macadamia Nuts					
6.	Pecans					
7.	Pistachio					
8.	Flax Seeds					
9.	Pumpkin Seeds					
10.	Sesame Seeds					
11.	Sunflower seeds					
12.	Walnuts					
Add your other favorite items below						
13.						
14.						
15.						
16.						

Table 8. Spices and herbs

#	Name	You	1	2	3	4
1.	Basil					
2.	Black pepper					
3.	Cinnamon					
4.	Garlic					
5.	Ginger					
6.	Mint					
7.	Oregano					
8.	Paprika					
9.	Parsley					
10.	Red pepper					
11.	Salt					
12.	Sea Salt					
Add your other favorite items below						
13.						
14.						
15.						
16.						

Table 9. Baked goods

#	Name	You	1	2	3	4
1.	Bagels					
2.	Buns					
3.	Cake					
4.	Cookies					
5.	Croissants					
6.	Donuts					
7.	Pastries					
8.	Pita bread					
9.	Rolls					
10.	Rye bread					
11.	Wheat Bread					
Add your other favorite items below						
12.						
13.						
14.						
15.						
16.						

Table 10. Condiments / Sauces

#	Name	You	1	2	3	4
1.	BBQ sauce					
2.	Honey					
3.	Hot sauce					
4.	Jam					
5.	Ketchup					
6.	Maple syrup					
7.	Mayonnaise					
8.	Mustard					
9.	Relish					
10.	Salsa					
11.	Soy sauce					
12.	Vinegar					
Add your other favorite items below						
13.						
14.						
15.						
16.						

Table 11. Drink list

#	Name	You	1	2	3	4
1.	Apple juice					
2.	Black tea					
3.	Carrot juice					
4.	Coffee					
5.	Grape juice					
6.	Green tea					
7.	Chamomile tea					
8.	Mint tea					
9.	Hot chocolate					
10.	Orange juice					
11.	Tomato juice					
12.	White tea					
Add your other favorite items below						
13.						
14.						
15.						
16.						

Table 12. Alcoholic beverage list

#	Name	You	1	2	3	4
1.	Beer					
2.	Brandy					
3.	Champagne					
4.	Gin					
5.	Red wine					
6.	Rum					
7.	Sake					
8.	Vodka					
9.	Whiskey					
10.	White wine					
Add your other favorite items below						
11.						
12.						
13.						
14.						
15.						

Table 13. Oils

#	Name	You	1	2	3	4
1.	Avocado oil					
2.	Almond oil					
3.	Canola oil					
4.	Coconut oil					
5.	Grapeseed oil					
6.	Macadamia oil					
7.	Olive oil					
8.	Sesame oil					
9.	Sunflower seed oil					
10.	Safflower oil					
11.	Palm oil					
12.	Walnut oil					
Add your other favorite items below						
13.						
14.						
15.						
16.						

Table 14. Your favorite foods

#	Name	You	1	2	3	4
Add your other favorite foods below						
1.						
2.						
3.						
4.						
5.						
6.						
7.						
8.						
9.						
10.						
11.						
12.						
13.						
14.						
15.						
16.						

Table 15. More your favorite foods

#	Name	You	1	2	3	4
Add your other favorite foods below						
1.						
2.						
3.						
4.						
5.						
6.						
7.						
8.						
9.						
10.						
11.						
12.						
13.						
14.						
15.						
16.						

Bibliography and Metaphysical Art

1. Donna Eden, David Feinstein, Energy Medicine, 2008.

2. Lee Carol's channeling of Kryon at:
https://www.kryon.com/k_freeaudio.html.

3. Lee Carol, The Recalibration of Humanity: 2013 and Beyond, 2013.

4. Ph.D. Mark G. Christensen (Author),   D.C., M.B.A. Martin W. Kollasch (Editor), JOB ANALYSIS OF CHI-ROPRACTIC 2005, ISBN 1-884457-05-3, 208 p. Publisher: NATIONAL BOARD OF CHIROPRACTIC EXAMINERS

5. Ellen W. Cutler, Winning the War against Immune Disorders & Allergies, 1998, 582 p.

6. John G. Ryan, The Missing Pill, 2013

7. Energized for healing guided 2 minutes Meditation for good effective sleep. Video by Alexander Khomoutov at:
https://www.youtube.com/watch?v=r1b1JvGiJCM

8. Opening to Love – metaphysical art print for love and good luck by Elena Khomoutova at:
http://lightfromart.com/node/8

9. Prosperity – metaphysical art print for prosperity and good luck by artist Elena Khomoutova at:
http://lightfromart.com/node/12

10. Roses for Love – metaphysical art print for love and good luck by Alexander Khomoutov at:
http://lightfromart.com/node/97

11. Leading-edge Healing group sessions, meditations: 16

hours audio downloads at:

http://lightfromart.com/node/121

12. <u>Dr. Alexander Khomoutov, Inspirational Healing Quotes: 52 Weeks to a More Joyful Life, Better Health and Motivation, 2017.</u>

13. <u>Dr. Alexander Khomoutov, O Canada! Discover Famous Canadian Cities and Landscapes in Art Paintings, Prints and Photographs, 2017.</u>

14. <u>Dr. Alexander Khomoutov, Choose the Joy of Art for Your Baby's Room! Bring Positive Healing Energy and Good Luck to Your Baby through Unique Wall Art, 2017.</u>

Dr. Alexander Khomoutov, Ph.D.

An extract from the full-length book
Choose the Joy of Art for Your Baby's Room!

Bring Positive Healing Energy and Good Luck to Your Baby through Unique Wall Art

Dr. Alexander Khomoutov, Ph.D.

The New Children are arriving and they bring with them many gifts of consciousness, knowledge and wisdom - gifts that will serve to change humanity in the most remarkable of ways. They thrive in balanced environments full of love and integrity. The time to foster this is with the newborn - and this wonderful book will show you how to do just that!

Thank you Alexander for creating a wonderful resource - full of tips and tools to help you create the perfect environment as you welcome this precious new life in your heart and your home!

Dr. John G. Ryan, MD

Specialist Medical Doctor, consciousness and energy based healer, University Professor, Author of The Missing Pill

This book explains how important it is to use positive energy pieces of artwork while decorating your infant's nursery. It shows you how to test the energy, as well as, determine the type of artwork that is best for you and your child. It is well written and filled with many suggestions to help create a loving, healing, and lucky environment for your child. I highly recommend it to young parents who want to create an energy balanced nursery to nurture their infant.

Dianne C. Nassr, L.C. M.S.W.

Energy healer and contributing author of A Juicy, Joyful Life: Inspiration from Women Who Have Found the Sweetness in Every Day.

Dedication

The book is dedicated to all of you who are open to discovering the power within yourselves to live a happy, joyful and healthy life ever after...

Table of Contents

Acknowledgments

Thank you to my wife, Elena, and my angel, Joy, for the inspiration. Elena, the first reader, gave me so many suggestions.

I'm so thankful to my parents, who gave me the freedom to do what I love. They always trusted that I would use this freedom in a very positive and loving way. Very special thanks to my mother who showed me how to use the greatest power within. In 1960s and70s she was already successfully using applied kinesiology – using a pendulum —to determine blood pressure and other things.

I'm very grateful to Lee Carroll and Kryon. Their teachings about the Innate have inspired me. They gave me a magic key to unlock the sacred door to my healing and joy.

I'd like to express my very special thanks to Dr. John G. Ryan, MD, whose book "The Missing Pill" gave me deeper understanding of Quantum DNA.

I'm so grateful to Dianne Nassr. Dianne taught me how to use the Sway test when I was hosting the "Healing with Lightworkers" telesummit. This is the main method I use now. She also gave me numerous suggestions to improve the book.

I'm so thankful to Janet Hofstetter for copy editing.

I'm sending you all my Love, Light and Hugs.

Alexander Khomoutov

Disclaimer

The author of this book does not dispense medical advice or prescribe the use of any technique as a form of diagnosis or treatment for physical, emotional or medical problems without advice of a physician, either directly or indirectly. The intent of the author is only to offer information of a general nature to help you in your quest for emotional and spiritual well-being.

Please also be informed that any artworks, images, information from this book, etc. are not intended to diagnose, treat, cure or prevent any condition, including: physical, financial or any other problems. The information received through any of these means should not in any way be used as a substitute for advice from a Medical Advisor or other licensed Professionals.

In the event you use any of the information in this book for yourself, the author and the publisher assume no responsibility for your actions.

Introduction

Do you want to discover how to choose artworks that bring positive healing energy to your baby?

Would you like to know how to find art paintings and prints that bring good luck to you and your baby?

Shhhh... Do you want to discover some SECRETS that the art industry doesn't want you to know and that could save you some money?

You're in a right place, because you find all in this book now...

You could use ideas from this book not only for your baby's room but for your other rooms too...

Your first step is to read this book in its entirety. Please don't just skim through it. I don't want you to miss a single word, because when I demystify the art of choosing artwork for you, you simply cannot fail to find artwork that brings positive energy to your baby.

So, how do you choose art for your baby's room?

Do you consider the following?

- The subject of the painting or print should be suitable for a baby's room.

- The main colors should be in harmony with the colors of the furniture in the room and the wallpaper or painted walls.

- The main colors of the artwork might be different for a baby girl's or boy's room.

You are right - all of those things are important. But have you considered what kind of energy the artwork brings to your baby?

Artwork can bring your baby negative, toxic energy or positive, healing energy. See fig.1. Even if two pieces of art have similar subjects, they could have opposite energies. Read on and you will learn several methods to help you choose artwork that will bring positive energy for healing and good luck to your baby. You will also learn how to avoid art with toxic energies.

You will discover how to choose museum quality giclee paper, canvas or embellished fine art prints for your nursery. Through the use of a comparison chart you will learn an easy way to choose an art print.

I have been working with art color printing for more than 15 years, so I can provide you with important insider information that will be useful to you in choosing the right artwork for your nursery.

You will discover in this book some secrets that the art industry doesn't want you to know. You will learn not only how to choose art that brings you and your baby positive energy, but you will learn some secrets that could save you money when you buy art. You will also discover some secrets about how to choose art prints that will bring you joy with beautiful colors for many years. Your grandchildren and their grandchildren can enjoy the beautiful colors in these art prints for many generations to come. You will also learn the important questions to ask before you buy an art print and how to save yourself from choosing art with colors that could fade away in just a few months.

So read on to discover more art secrets and tips and find out why I started to print art myself instead of hiring some printing company.

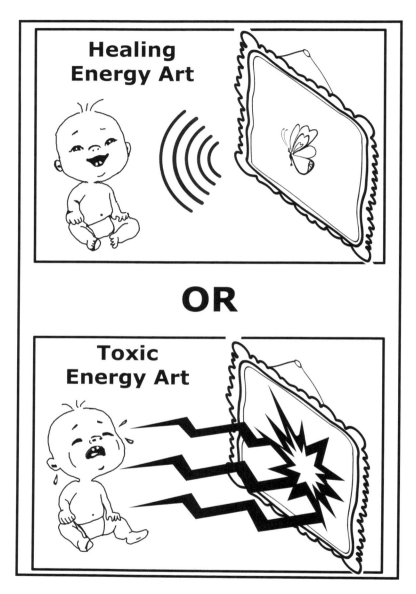

Fig.1. Artwork can bring your baby positive healing energy or negative toxic energy.

1. How to choose fine art that brings positive healing energy and good luck to your baby

When you visit an art gallery or an art exhibit, do you find that some paintings bring you joy and you could look at them for a long time? Do you find that other paintings give you uncomfortable sensations, even though they might have a pleasant subject and beautiful colors? In these two scenarios, you are feeling energy related to the artist's intent.

According to art research [1] the artist's energy is transferred to the artwork during creation. We feel this energy when we look at it. In some cases, it can bring healing. For example, according to medical research some of Nicholas Roerich's paintings bring healing to the observers. S. Smirnov investigated the art painting "The Last Day of Pompeii" by Karl Bryullov [1, 2]. The subject of the painting is tragic but the painting emanates positive energy. So the energy of the artist's intention is very important. In some cases, the subject of the artwork is positive, but it brings negative energy to anyone who spends time gazing at it. So it's very important to find artwork that will bring positive energy, joy and good luck to your baby.

Several methods are available to find out what kind of energy an artwork will bring to your baby:

- The artist's intention method

- The heart method

- The enhanced heart method, which combines artist's intention and heart methods

- The applied kinesiology methods

1.1 The artist's intention method

Let's say you found some artworks that you like. Try using the artist's intention method first. Before making your decision, do some internet research to find out more about the type of art you are looking for and the artist who created it. To understand the artist's intention in general, visit the artist's website and read the artist's statement.

What do you think about the following artist's statement?

Do you want more good luck, happiness, love, healing and rejuvenation? Then metaphysical positive energy art paintings, paper or canvas art prints, healing books by Ottawa artists and authors are for you.

Yes, you are right, the artist's intention is to bring you positive energy and good luck through the art. Then what is the next step? Explore artworks on the artist's website and find some that you like. After that, read the story about each one that you have chosen and find out what the artist's intention was while he or she created it.

What do you think about the following artist's intention for a particular art painting?

> *Artist's intention: To create art to help you in discovering and using the amazing power within yourself to bring you joy, good luck and...*

While examining artworks, you may find some that look very promising. Find another one by the same artist and see if both of them were created to bring positive energy, then choose the one that you like more.

If you are just starting your search for the art, copy the above whole artist statement or the artist intention and paste it as your internet search. You will find the positive energy art images. Then choose the one you like most. That's it.

I was planning to show you real examples of art and artists' statements that emanate a negative energy. I found such artworks. When I opened the web pages I immediately felt uncomfortable sensations and I even developed a headache. My only wish was to close those webpages at once. So I decided that my book will focus only on positive energy art.

Sometimes, big gallery websites do not have enough information about their paintings or artists, so it's not easy to make a decision. In this case, search for the artists' own websites to find out more about them and understand their intentions.

What if you find an artist who hasn't provided that kind of statement? Try to find the artist's biographical information to learn more about the artist's intention.

If you still can't discover the artist's intention, read on to find other methods that could help you in these cases.

1.2 The heart method

If you find some artwork that you like, but you can't find any artist's statements of intentions, try using the heart method.

Use the following steps to use the heart method:

9. Go to a quiet room free of distractions like music or television.

   For me, it works best when I'm alone in the room, but you could do it with somebody else who is willing to do it with you.

10. Stand still or sit down in your favorite chair.

11. Let go of all worries and relax your body. If you are comfortable doing so, close your eyes. If you find it difficult to do with your eyes closed, doing it with your eyes open is OK too.

12. Put your right hand on your chest at your heart area.

13. Take 3 deep breaths, focusing your attention on your heart area.

14. Ask aloud "Dear heart! Does <title of the artwork you are checking, for example: "Multidimensional Eternal Bliss"> bring me and my baby positive energy and good luck? Thank you".

15. Sense what you feel. Do you have some pleasant comfortable sensations, maybe even goosebumps? Then the answer is Yes. Otherwise the answer is No.

To practice this method, say aloud statements about something that you know is 100% true, for example, "Dear heart! My name is <your name>. Thank you". In my case, I say "Dear heart! My name is Alexander. Thank you".

Then, sense what you feel. You could have some unique sensations. Remember them. Then, when you ask the question about the artwork, notice whether you have similar sensations indicating that the answer is YES.

Try asking aloud something that you know that is 100% false, for example, "Dear heart! My name is <somebody's name>. Thank you". In my case, I say "Dear heart! My name is Elena. Thank you".

Then sense what you feel. Remember the sensations. When you ask questions about artwork and you have similar sensations, the answer is No.

The more you practice this technique, the more reliable it becomes.

1.3 The enhanced heart method

If you are using the artist's intention method and you are still not sure what kind of energy the artwork will bring to you and your baby, add the artist's intention and the heart methods together. I call it the enhanced heart method.

Using this method you could have more reliable results. This is especially true when you are buying prints that are not created by the artist themselves. Sometimes they are mass-produced using cheap labor to make art prints cheaper. Do you know what kind of energy this process will add? I don't know either. So the first method could fail if you will rely solely on it. The enhanced heart method will give you more reliable answers.

If you could buy prints printed by the artists themselves, then you could use the artist's intention method, which is the best option.

For example, we print all our limited-edition prints ourselves and send them directly to our customers. In this case, we ensure quality and the energy of artwork remains intact in the prints. However, if you can't buy directly from the artist, another option is to buy prints done by local companies on behalf of the artist.

The more you practice, the more reliable your answers will be. Does this method work for everybody? For some people it will work just fine. For others it will not. For me, I've found that the most reliable method is the Applied Kinesiology method. I'm also using it in my healing practice. I wrote a book about it - "Heal Yourself" [3].

Read on and you will find more about Applied Kinesiology methods. Every person is unique, so find the method that is most reliable for you and use it. The more you use it, the more reliable your results.

1.4 Quantum methods

In sections 1.1 to 1.3 I explained how to choose fine art to bring positive healing energy and good luck to your baby's room. If you want to open your heart to learn new quantum ways of choosing art, keep reading! Quantum methods can be used not only to find out the energy of artworks, but also in your personal healing, and in many other aspects of your life...

Choose the Joy of Art for Your Baby's Room

Bring Positive Healing Energy and Good Luck to Your Baby through Unique Wall Art

Buy it:

US: www.amazon.com/dp/B07486VBF2

UK: www.amazon.co.uk/dp/B07486VBF2

Canada: www.amazon.ca/dp/B07486VBF2

You could use ideas from this book not only for your baby's room but for your other rooms too...

Heal Yourself!

Dr. Alexander Khomoutov, Ph.D.

An extract from the full-length book
Inspirational Healing Quotes:
52 Weeks to a More Joyful Life, Better Health and Motivation

When you are on the path of a spiritual messenger you understand the basic underlying principle that governs the law of creation and specifically, "how to create your life consciously" is this: "You create your life by the simple 3-step process of THOUGHT, WORD & DEED." Alexander Khomoutov has taken this foundational truth and put it into book form with his latest book, "Inspirational Healing Quotes".

This book may seem simple in concept and form but underlying this simplicity are profound truths and ways of being that transcend day to day living and will take you to a higher level of consciousness that not only allows you to be a better person but also affects all of humanity. My suggestion is to please take the time to fully engage in each quote for a full week and immerse yourself in the message so that it becomes a habit of living your life. That is my plan and I thank Alexander for this amazing opportunity and the platform of this book to do so.

If you truly desire to change your life in powerful positive ways then you must not only read this book for the Thoughts and the Words but then also take the Actions of using the quotes every week for the next 52 weeks. It will change your life in dramatic, positive and powerful ways.

Richard D. Blackstone

Award-winning author and international speaker about life, love and the true nature of how the universe works, Author of Nuts & Bolts Spirituality, and Waking up the Sleepwalkers.

While reading this book you'll find that Alexander has chosen some very inspirational quotes that will allow you to begin your day with amazing new positive energy. These quotes will encourage you to allow the energy of the quote to affect your life. The topics include joy, happiness, abundance and optimism. Focusing on one quote per week will enable you to shift your energy for the entire week. This will help develop this feeling of deserving and worthiness of joy, happiness, and abundance in your life. I recommend this book for anyone seeking a direction on how to improve their thoughts allowing the energy to ultimately improve their lifestyle. It is a wonderful addition to Alexander's other books!

Dianne C. Nassr, L.C. M.S.W.

Energy healer and contributing author of A Juicy, Joyful Life: Inspiration from Women Who Have Found the Sweetness in Every Day.

Dedication

The book is dedicated to all of you who are open to discovering the power within yourselves to live a happy, joyful and healthy life ever after...

Table of Contents

Acknowledgments

Thank you to my wife, Elena, and my angel, Joy, for the inspiration. Elena, the first reader, gave me so many suggestions.

I'm so thankful to my parents, who gave me the freedom to do what I love. They always trusted that I would use this freedom in a very positive and loving way. Very special thanks to my mother who showed me how to use the greatest power within.

I'm so thankful to Janet Hofstetter for copy editing.

I'm sending you all my Love, Light and Hugs☺.

Alexander Khomoutov

Disclaimer

The author of this book does not dispense medical advice or prescribe the use of any technique as a form of diagnosis or treatment for physical, emotional or medical problems without advice of a physician, either directly or indirectly. The intent of the author is only to offer information of a general nature to help you in your quest for emotional and spiritual well-being.

Please also be informed that any artworks, images, information from this book, etc. are not intended to diagnose, treat, cure or prevent any condition, including: physical, financial or any other problems. The information received through any of these means should not in any way be used as a substitute for advice from a Medical Advisor or other licensed Professionals.

In the event you use any of the information in this book for yourself, the author and the publisher assume no responsibility for your actions.

While the author made every effort to correctly attribute each quote to the original author, sometimes the origin is unknown.
The author has made every effort to verify internet addresses and other contact information at the time of publication, however he does not have any control over and does not assume any responsibility for third-party websites or their content.

Introduction

Do you want to start your healing now?

Do you want to bring positive energy to your life?

Do you want to have the wisdom of the ages at your fingertips?

You're in a right place, because this book gives you the instant access to wisdom of the ages and joyful artworks that were created with the intention to bring healing and good luck to you.

This is not just a book of quotations - it's a tool for bringing you positive energy for healing, good luck, and love. Use it to unlock the miraculous power within you to live a healthy, happy and joyful life.

Your first step is to read this book in its entirety. Please don't just skim through it. I don't want you to miss a single word, because each page and each artwork bring positive healing energy to you.

One of the effective ways to use this book is the following:

- There are 52 quotes in the book. First, read the book from the beginning, then read just one quote a week in any order.

- Live this quote for the whole week! Put it into action. Allow this quote to be your inspiration. Write it down and keep it with you. Read it at least twice a day.

- Choose a different quote each week and so on for 52 weeks

- Open your heart to the positive energy of quotes and accompanying pictures. Trust the process. Enjoy the results and be grateful for the outcome.

An artwork can bring you positive, healing energy. Find more about it in my book *Choose the Joy of Art for Your Baby's Room!* [1].

I have created healing art prints using some of the quotes from this book. To get a print of your favorite picture and quote, visit www.LightFromArt.com [2]. Put the print on your wall. Act on a quote and enjoy positive energy of the artwork.

Thank you for choosing my book. I'm sending you my Love, Light and Hugs☺.

Inspirational Healing Quotes:
52 Weeks to a More Joyful Life, Better Health and Motivation

Buy it:

US: www.amazon.com/dp/B077PK5J3H
UK: http://www.amazon.co.uk/dp/B077PK5J3H
Canada: www.amazon.ca/dp/B077PK5J3H

GET YOUR 7 FREE GIFTS

I create my artworks, photographs and books with the intention of bringing you healing energy and good luck.

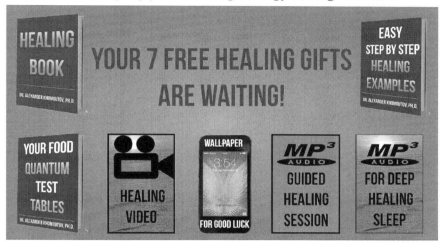

Building a relationship with you my readers is the greatest thing about writing. I occasionally send information to my Readers Group about new healing ideas and new healing books releases. You'll be the first to know next time I have some cool stuff to give away or other special offers!

Join my Reader's Group and I'll send you all this stuff FOR FREE:

1. Easy step by step healing examples: How I heal myself, my wife and more... Exclusive to my Readers Group mailing list – you can't get this anywhere else.
2. Healing book - PDF file.
3. Healing video.
4. For deep healing sleep - Audio MP3 file. Exclusive to my Readers Group.

5. New good luck energy wallpaper for your iPhone/Android or other smartphone.
6. A great healing session —audio MP3 file (about 1 hour recording).
7. Your Food Quantum Test Tables - PDF file.

Get 7 healing gifts for FREE, when you sign up for my Reader's Group.

Click here to get started:

www.LightFromArt.com/gifts

Other resources

Find out about metaphysical energy art designed to help you in your first conversations with your Quantum DNA at:

www.LightFromArt.com

Listen to Lee Carol's channeling of Kryon at:

https://www.kryon.com/k_freeaudio.html

Visit Dr. John Ryan's website at:

http://drjohnryan.org

Visit energy healer Dianne Nassr's website at:

http://diannenassr.com/

Check out Dianne Nassr's article in the following book:

A Juicy, Joyful Life: Inspiration from Women Who Have Found the Sweetness in Every Day, by Linda Joy, 2010.

Watch 5 minutes of Donna Eden's energy exercises at:

https://www.youtube.com/watch?v=gffKhttrRw4

Check out spiritual metaphysical energy art prints designed for good luck, love, and healing at:

http://lightfromart.com/catalog/3

Discover spiritual metaphysical art cards for good luck at:

http://lightfromart.com/node/110

Discover Healing with audio group sessions, meditations: 16 hours audio downloads from Healing with Lightworkers telesummit at:

http://lightfromart.com/node/121

Check out positive energy art cards designed for good luck:

http://charitycards.ca/christmas-greeting-card-rtists/elena_khomoutova/

http://charitycards.ca/christmas-greeting-card-artists/alex_khomoutov/

http://www2.editionsdevillers.com/commerce/elena-khomoutova

http://www2.editionsdevillers.com/commerce/alexander-khomoutov

Check out Marcy Rae Lifavi's book: Eletunji, The Shiny Elephant: A Fable: Spiritual and Psychological Journey Creates Choice for A Nurturing Voice at:

https://www.amazon.com/dp/B00QXYTBLQ

Healing Art

It's not just art - it's a metaphysical energy art tool for healing, good luck, love and unlocking the miraculous power within you to live a healthy, happy and joyful life. It's created to ease up your connection to your Quantum DNA for your healing and...

Discover more at:

www.lightfromart.com

Connect with Alexander

Thank you very much for taking the time to read this book. I'm excited for you to start your path to healing and to live a healthy, happy and joyful life.

If you have any questions, feel free to contact me at: www.lightfromart.com/contact

You could follow me on Twitter: @_Alex_K

Become a fan and have a fun at:

www.facebook.com/LightFromArt

You can check out my blog for the latest updates here:

www.lightfromart.com/blog

I'm wishing you the best of health, happiness and success!

Sending you LIGHT and LOVE☺.

Alexander Khomoutov

About the Author

Dr. Alexander Khomoutov holds a Ph.D. in Building Physics. He has a great passion for writing, photography, and healing art. Alexander creates his artworks, photographs and books with the intention of bringing you quantum healing energy and good luck. He also enjoys hiking, tennis, skiing and sending Light. His angels, wife Elena and their budgie Joy, are inspirations for Alexander's creations. Joy often sneaks into his pockets or even under his shirt and... makes him laugh ☺.

Discover more at:

www.lightfromart.com/Dr-AK-books

Get free healing videos and gifts from Alexander at:

www.LightFromArt.com/gifts

Other books by Dr. Alexander Khomoutov Ph.D.

Inspirational Healing Quotes: 52 Weeks to a More Joyful Life, Better Health and Motivation.

Do you want to start your healing now?

Would you like to bring positive energy to your life?

Are you ready to have the wisdom of the ages at your fingertips?

You're in a right place, because Inspirational Healing Quotes book gives you the instant access to wisdom of the ages and joyful artworks that were created with the intention to bring healing and good luck to you.

This is not just a book of quotations - it's a tool for bringing you positive energy for healing, good luck, and love. Use it to unlock the miraculous power within you to live a healthy, happy and joyful life.

Get it:

US: www.amazon.com/dp/B077PK5J3H

UK: http://www.amazon.co.uk/dp/B077PK5J3H

Canada: www.amazon.ca/dp/B077PK5J3H

Choose the Joy of Art for Your Baby's Room! Bring Positive Healing Energy and Good Luck to Your Baby through Unique Wall Art

Do you want to discover how to choose artworks that bring positive healing energy to your baby?

Would you like to know how to find art paintings and prints that bring good luck to you and your baby?

Shhhh... Do you want to discover some SECRETS that the art industry doesn't want you to know and that could save you some money?

You're in a right place, because you find all in this book now...

You could use ideas from this book not only for your baby's room but for your other rooms too...

Buy it:

US: www.amazon.com/dp/B07486VBF2

UK: www.amazon.co.uk/dp/B07486VBF2

Canada: www.amazon.ca/dp/B07486VBF2

O Canada! Discover Famous Canadian Cities and Landscapes in Art Paintings, Prints and Photographs

Are you ready to discover famous Canadian cities and landscapes?

Would you like to enjoy legendary Canadian Rockies, Maligne Lake and more...?

Do you want to see how Canadians celebrate winter holidays?

You are in the right place now, because this book gives you an instant joy with 73 fine artworks and photos!

Your first step is to read this book in its entirety. Don't miss a single page, because each one was created with intention to bring positive energy and joy to you.

In this book, you will find images of art paintings and photographs of well-known places in Canada, including Ottawa, Quebec City, Montreal, Mont Tremblant, Vancouver, Victoria, Canadian Rockies and more...

Buy it:

US: www.amazon.com/dp/B0739PW36C

UK: www.amazon.co.uk/dp/B0739PW36C

Canada: www.amazon.ca/dp/B0739PW36C

Heal Yourself! 3 Easy Steps to Discovering and Using Your Quantum Healing Energy.

Concise Edition

Do you want to discover how to heal yourself? You're in the right place, because these easy effective 3 steps take only few minutes to learn now and can be used instantly!

This is a concise edition of my book, Heal Yourself! It includes core information for communicating with your spiritual (or quantum) DNA, including the basic "Sway" method.

Get it:

US: www.amazon.com/dp/B07492FNGQ

UK: http://www.amazon.co.uk/dp/B07492FNGQ

Canada: www.amazon.ca/dp/B07492FNGQ

More books coming soon. You can sign up to be notified of new releases, giveaways and pre-release specials - plus, get 7 free gifts at:

www.LightFromArt.com/gifts

Find an updated list of new books by Alexander at:

www.lightfromart.com/Dr-AK-books

One More Thing...

Thank you for reading! If you've enjoyed this book or found it useful I would be very grateful if you'd post a short review on the book's Amazon page.

You can jump right to the page by clicking below.

US: www.amazon.com/dp/B0749C5HCJ

UK: www.amazon.co.uk/dp/B0749C5HCJ

Canada: www.amazon.ca/dp/B0749C5HCJ

Your support really does make a difference and I read all the reviews personally so I can get your feedback and make my books even better.

Thank you very much for your support!

Alexander Khomoutov

Put your healing plan below!

Heal Yourself!

39171537R00083

Made in the USA
Lexington, KY
16 May 2019